Illness
& Healing

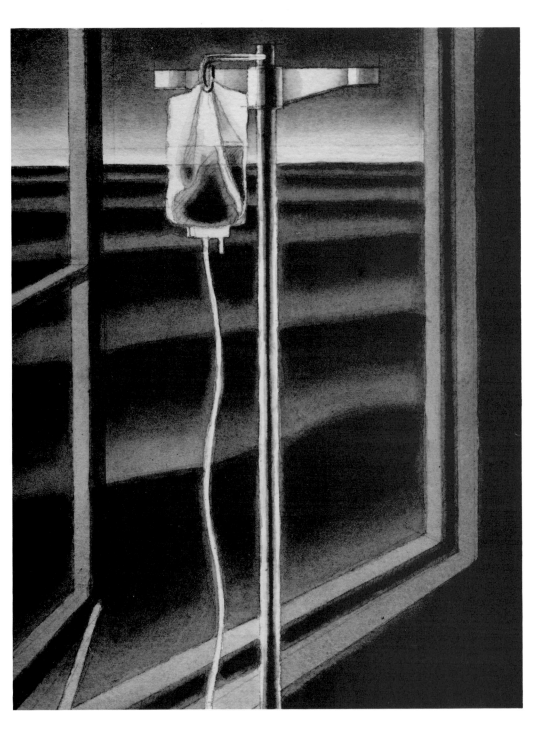

Illness & Healing

Images of Cancer
by Robert Pope

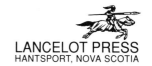

LANCELOT PRESS
HANTSPORT, NOVA SCOTIA

ISBN 0-88999-480-3
Published 1991
Second printing January 1995
Third printing January 1997
Fourth printing January 1999

LANCELOT PRESS LIMITED
Hantsport, Nova Scotia
Office and production facilities situated on
Highway No. 1, 1/2 mile east of Hantsport.

MAILING ADDRESS
P.O. Box 425, Hantsport, N.S. B0P 1P0

Front Cover:
Hug, 1990 (detail)
Acrylic on canvas, 182.9 x 78.7 cm

Frontispiece (page 2)
Intravenous Solution and Ocean, 1991
Acrylic on paper, 24.5 x 19.1 cm

Back Cover:
Sparrow, 1989
Acrylic on canvas, 61.0 x 76.2 cm

Dedication

This book is dedicated to my family,

to Ross Langley and Wayne Diotte who are
two healers instrumental in my recovery
and continuing health,

and to all cancer patients everywhere.

Contents

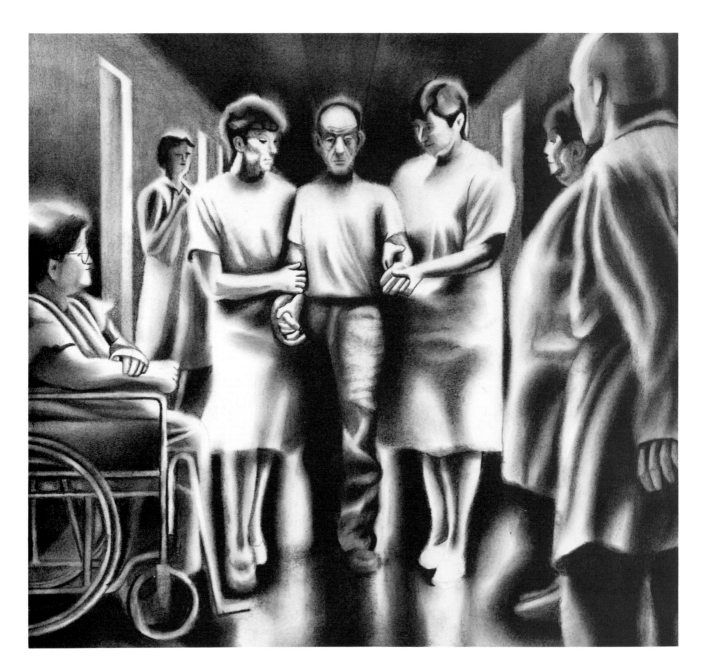

Foreword by Ross Langley, M.D.

There will be few who examine the paintings in this book who will not be moved. Those patients and families who have faced cancer will likely be reminded of their personal experience, as they witness how one determined young man comes to terms with a decade-long ordeal.

I've never asked but rather assumed that Robert Pope's purpose in this series of paintings was to depict for all of us, patients, families, physicians, and friends, what actually happens during the diagnosis, treatment and recovery from a life-threatening illness. For students of medicine this book will rightfully take its place with such classic narratives as that of Daisy Tagliacozzo and Hans Mauksch in 1972, describing the human side of medicine and from a patient's perspective. Both tell us not what we would like to hear or see, but what we ought to know.

The sciences and the humanities should work hand in hand in the care of the sick. Often they do not. And sometimes there is just not enough of either, in spite of everyone's best efforts. We owe to our colleagues in scientific research the knowledge and technology that has so improved the scientific care of the patient in modern times. Although a "New Humanism" movement began around the turn of this century, only in the last 20 years, through the efforts of Pellegrino and others, was the mutual impoverishment of the humanities and medicine realized, and also the particular need for research into, and continuing application of, the humanities in medicine. Robert Pope's research into the human condition contributes to that thrust. We can be grateful to him, to the Canada Council, the patients and institutions in Halifax and Toronto which supported him, for the results.

Opposite:
New Steps, 1990
Charcoal on paper, 34.7 x 39.0 cm

9

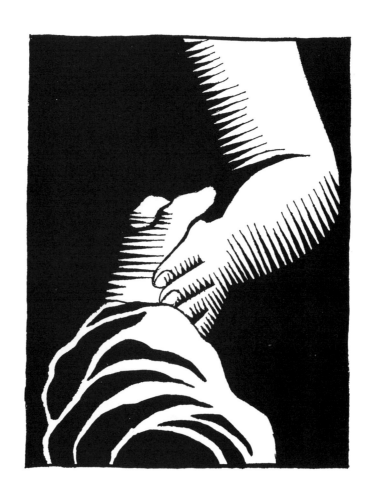

Holding Hands, 1991
Ink on paper, 11.4 x 8.8 cm

Introduction by Jean Cameron

This book is a vivid, powerful, and unflinching look at the lived and re-lived experiences of one man's battle with cancer.

In a way it could be said to be every cancer patient's story. Robert Pope describes the disease as brutal, ugly, and mean and its treatment "a living hell."

Through written words and pictures we share the total suffering: physical, emotional, social, and spiritual. But always there is the unspoken courage of the man, an artist and writer. To read the book is to be deeply moved.

In a way that words alone could never convey we move through the various stages of diagnosis and treatment, times of remission, dashed hopes, the awful necessity to go through it all again, and then, the calm of healing.

The cold impersonal aspects of hospital treatment are dramatically illustrated: the waiting line of wheelchairs that he likens to a factory assembly line; the lady who becomes a "piece of film"; the radiotherapy treatment rooms that are identified with the world of science fiction. We share the dehumanizing aspects of it all.

And then, in contrast, Robert Pope shows us the all too close human contacts with strangers. There are times when one needs and longs for privacy. It is easy to feel humiliated, being sick in public, and having to live all the most intimate and private aspects of life and death in public view.

But always there are the people who are close and special in life. The ones who are there through all the ups and downs. He recognizes the enormous importance of these human relationships. He reveals their complexities. He knows and conveys to us the strengthening and healing power of love and he expresses it in the most tender and poignant tribute to his mother.

In *Illness and Healing* the painful needles, relentless nausea and vomiting, the times when one simply "wants to die," the power and vulnerability of doctors, all hallmarks of cancer treatments, are laid before us, vividly expressed.

And yet, one has the sense that Robert Pope has been able to move inwardly away from all the suffering. He has distanced himself in a way that has enabled him to perceive even more clearly. He recognizes and reveals the presence of spiritual and religious symbols. He has been able to transform experiences into creative form.

When he looks out through the window of his hospital room one feels that he is perhaps realizing the beauty of nature as never before. But this looking out is not an escape or a wish to escape from the weakness and the pain. Rather it is an affirmation of his oneness with life in all its forms and conditions. He is not separated by his predicament. He is a part of it all and for him, the blossoms and the trees, that fragile bird, those high mountains are all strong symbols of hope and survival. He shares these gifts with all who see and read his book.

Dr. Viktor Frankl has told us that by our own attitude it is possible to transform even the most seemingly hopeless situations into achievement. I believe Robert Pope has done this. His courage and his attitude to what may have been the most painful and difficult experiences of his life are a measure of his own fulfillment as a human being.

Jean Cameron has worked in the palliative care unit of Royal Victoria Hospital in Montreal, and now makes her home in Phillipsburg, Quebec. She is the author of *Time to Live, Time to Die* which has been published in several languages.

Acknowledgements

I thank Dr. Ross Langley for his medical treatment and advice, for writing the foreword, and for his invaluable help in almost every aspect of this project. My appreciation goes out to the following nurses at the Victoria General Hospital: Gloria Repetto, Janet Copeland, and all the nurses on 8-West; and Sandy Redden and her staff on 4-A. As well, I offer my gratitude to the following people associated with the Victoria General: Chris Hansen at Public Relations, Chaplain Ed Fiander, Dr. Drew Bethune, Dr. Audley Bodurtha, Dr. George Carruthers, Dr. Fred Wilms and Dr. Vanora Haldane. To Tia Cooper and Annette Penny at the Izaak Walton Killam Hospital; Dr. Emerson Moffitt and Harry Churchill at the Cancer Treatment and Research Foundation; and Katherine Miner, Leslie Dutton and Dr. Simon Sutcliffe at the Princess Margaret Hospital, my thanks.

Many people served as models for these pictures. I am indebted to all the patients, too numerous to mention, at the various hospitals I visited. Also, too great in number to mention individually, are the friends who posed for me, and the friends who offered useful criticism and comments.

I am grateful to the Canada Council for two one-year grants which funded this work. To Jean Cameron for her introduction and kind words, my thanks. Mern O'Brien and Susan Gibson-Garvey at the Dalhousie Art Gallery, and Ineke Felderhof-Graham at Studio 21 were very helpful. As well, I appreciate Horst Deppe's design advice.

Finally, I thank my family: my brother Doug for providing the spark to get this book underway, my sister Janet and mother Isabel for their suggestions and support, and my dad Bill in his capacity as publisher.

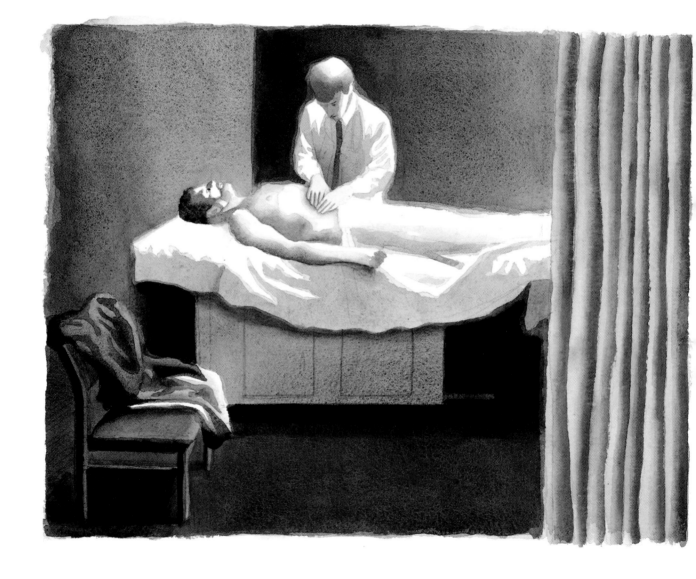

1

Personal Experience

It was on an unimaginably beautiful spring morning that I noticed my first sign of cancer. The sun was streaming in the bathroom window through the curtains and I was standing over the sink shaving when I noticed a lump on my neck. Amazingly, it was about one half the size of a golf ball. I knew that something was wrong.

This slowly developed into a sense that something was terribly wrong. I remember sitting across the desk from my busy family doctor. He didn't seem too concerned as he referred me to a specialist. The specialist was much more tense as he told me I would be admitted to hospital for tests. Although he didn't tell me, he knew I had cancer as soon as he saw me.

During the weeks of diagnosis in the hospital I still didn't know what was wrong with me. I remember coming out of general anesthetic. Two friends, out of focus and shimmering above me, were making jokes it hurt to laugh at. I remember standing with a bathrobe on in the hallway talking to my parents on a pay phone. My brother brought me a collection of Dostoyevsky stories. I had brief visits from distant-seeming doctors. Nurses took my blood pressure and temperature regularly, and I found myself liking and admiring them.

Opposite:
Abdominal Examination, 1989
Acrylic on paper, 24.0 x 34.0 cm

15

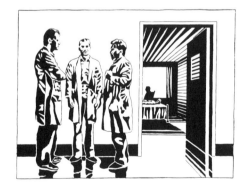

An endless parade of technicians came by for blood tests or to take me for x-rays or various scans. A large portion of my day was spent lying underneath machines.

Finally, feeling quite frustrated, I asked my doctors if they would tell me exactly what my illness was. They told me I had an advanced state of Hodgkin's disease, a cancer of the lymphatic system. Lymph nodes in my neck, under my armpits, in my groin, and other areas were cancerous. The cause of it is unknown. They told me it is one of the most curable cancers and even though I was in a late stage, I had about a 75% chance of being completely cured. Chemotherapy would start the next day.

The preceding weeks had to some degree prepared me for this news and the hope of being cured softened the blow. Still the word "cancer" is so loaded that it alone has a devastating effect. The main emotion I felt was numbness. How are you to feel when a stranger tells you that you have cancer? The numbness continued as I directed most of my thoughts to the mysterious treatment which would be starting disorientingly soon. When an expert in a white coat tells you there is a 25% chance you will die, it produces a very, very uncomfortable feeling. The night before the treatment started I had fifteen visitors sitting around my bed. I wasn't sure if I was at a party or a wake.

The word "chemotherapy" is short for chemical therapy. I received a combination of four drugs called MOPP. The "M" stands for nitrogen mustard, the main ingredient in mustard gas used in chemical warfare. Modern medicine was about to wage war inside my body. Two drugs were injected into my arm by syringe, and two I took in pill form. I was on a fourteen-day cycle with pills every day and injections on day one and day eight. I would then have fourteen days off. The complete treatment takes about six months.

It was late afternoon when a nurse brought in a tray loaded with syringes and bottles of chemicals. At four o'clock a doctor wearing gloves came to perform the injection. It took about ten minutes to push all the drugs into my arm. I felt a burning sensation in my vein and noticed a metallic taste in my mouth. Afterwards I sat with my father in the lounge. The problems of the beautiful people in the soap opera on the television seemed very different from my own.

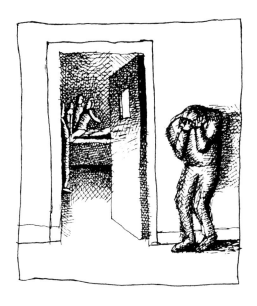

In chemotherapy, the drugs enter the bloodstream and destroy cancer cells. Unfortunately, they also destroy some healthy cells, causing side effects, including sterility. With each treatment, the side effects became worse until they began to overshadow everything, even my illness. My whole life revolved around injection days. I would vomit continuously for five hours and then spend two or three days afterwards slightly less but still severely nauseated. Because the chemotherapy was destroying normal blood cells, sometimes my blood count would drop to dangerously low levels and the injections would have to be delayed for days or weeks.

It was difficult to struggle through this period. The two things that helped me the most were family support and the hope of a cure. Finally, after seven months, the MOPP treatment was completed and all the tests were repeated. I felt like a student awaiting an exam result or a defendant about to hear the verdict from a jury.

The tests showed that the cancer was gone and I was considered in complete remission. This condition was short-lived, however, and four months later the cancer reappeared in my neck. The doctors immediately suggested repeating another six months of chemotherapy with four different and "better" drugs. Chances of a cure were lessened, but still good. I reluctantly agreed. Just before injecting the first of the

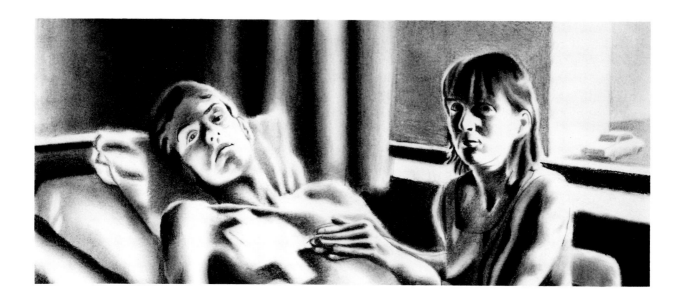

Above:
Surgery, 1990 (detail)
Charcoal on paper, 32.9 x 37.2 cm

Opposite:
Progress, 1990
Charcoal on paper, 40.6 x 27.0 cm

new drugs the doctor assured me that I wouldn't be sick this time. I wanted to believe him but I knew he was lying.

This was the worst period of my life. Any conception of hell I had paled next to what I was living through. I was weakened from the first course of chemotherapy and the side effects were even more severe. There were times when I was in so much pain from the treatments that I felt like dying. My family literally had to force me to go to the hospital for injections. My blood counts dropped lower and again I had treatment delays. I had fewer visits from friends and came to realize that one of the consequences of cancer was feeling alone.

With great difficulty the second course of chemotherapy was eventually completed. Again I was considered in remission, and again the cancer returned a few months later. Six months after the end of chemotherapy I waited in the doctor's office for the latest test results. I was beyond nervousness as I looked down over the beautiful, tree-covered city. The doctor didn't waste any words or give me much hope. There was cancer in my neck and in my abdomen. The only option remaining was to give radiation treatments to the areas where the cancer could be seen. Things were extremely serious. I was now given a 20% chance of living.

I sat in my apartment looking at a white wall. I had reached a turning point. The doctor's frankness had stripped away what was left of any protective numbness I may still have felt. I was facing death and I felt afraid. I looked at the white wall some more and decided on two courses of action. First, I would go through the radiation treatments and, second, I would try to assume some responsibility for my own healing and look into alternate therapies. I would do all I could while I still had the strength.

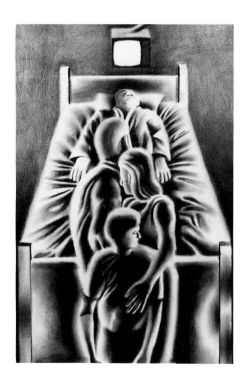

Whereas chemotherapy enters the bloodstream and goes throughout the body, radiation therapy consists of x-rays directed to specific parts. Because cancer cells do not exist totally independent of normal cells, the beams of radiation that kill cancer also damage nearby healthy tissues. Every day in the treatment room I would be positioned on a table which reminded me of an altar. Above me was a large machine which produced the rays of radiation. I received three or four minutes of exposure on the front and the same on the back. I felt like I was in an apocalyptic tanning salon.

I received forty radiation treatments in total: twenty to my neck and chest and twenty to my abdomen. The side effects were nausea, loss of appetite, tiredness, and lowered blood counts. These treatments permanently destroyed two-thirds of my bone marrow. The main concern of the doctors was the possibility of missing any cancer cells with the radiation. If only one cancer cell

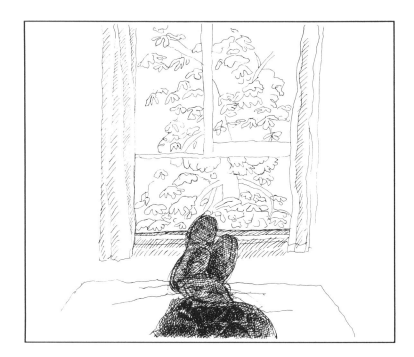

This page:
Chestnut Tree, 1986
Ink on paper, 27.8 x 35.6 cm

Opposite:
New Field, 1991
Ink on board, 14.5 x 18.0 cm

remained in the body, the treatments would fail. I could not have made it through those months of radiation without the presence and support of my family and friends.

After all the sincere, best efforts of modern medicine, my doctor gave me a 20% chance of living, a disquietingly small percentage that forced me to begin looking for alternatives to supplement the conventional therapy. I wanted something that didn't have bad side effects, was inexpensive, and that I could do myself.

Just at this moment, a friend lent me a book, *Recalled By Life*, by Anthony Sattilaro, M.D. In gripping, almost novelistic fashion Dr. Sattilaro describes how he cured his terminal prostate cancer by adopting something called a macrobiotic diet. The idea of treating illness with food seemed to be both radical and good common sense. Within days of reading this book I was on a plane bound for a macrobiotic centre in Boston. During a week of intensive cooking lessons, I realized that macrobiotics is more than a diet. Based on oriental philosophy and traditional wisdom, it is a wholistic approach that recognizes that every aspect of lifestyle is related to health.

This led me to practice a number of natural treatments for both mind and body, and I still follow most of this program. My diet consists of natural whole foods: 50% whole grains, 30% vegetables, 10% beans and sea vegetables, 5% soup and a few additional foods such as fruit, seeds, and fish. I eat no red meat, dairy products, sugar or chemicals. Basically, my diet includes

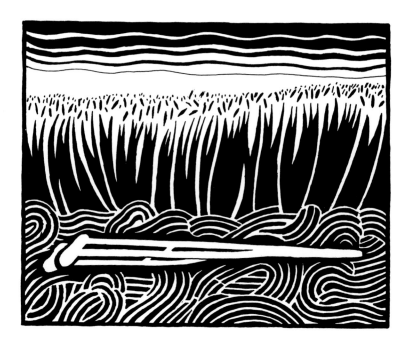

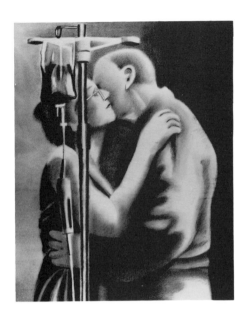

Hug 1, 1990
Charcoal on paper, 40.5 x 32.6 cm

foods that promote health and are known to prevent cancer and excludes foods that don't promote health and are known to increase chances of cancer. I exercise daily: fifteen minutes of stretching and self-massage each morning and evening, and an hour of walking each day.

I have learned that how you breathe can affect your health, and began to breathe more deeply. I began to use visualization and relaxation techniques to utilize the power of my mind against my disease. I changed my lifestyle to reduce stress. I concentrated on resolving unsatisfactory relationships. I made friends with others who were interested in natural approaches to healing. I was building a healthier life and this gave me a great feeling of empowerment. I began to feel much better.

More than five years have passed since my last radiation treatment, with no sign of cancer. My blood counts are still low but I am leading a normal, active life. I live with the knowledge that my cancer may recur or that the treatments I took may themselves cause new cancers. It is not easy to think about this, yet paradoxically, it helps me to go on. As Doctor Samuel Sanes, who died of cancer, has noted, the cancer patient observes two birthdays: the most important being the anniversary of his or her diagnosis, marking the years of survival. Living in the shadow of cancer makes every daily action an affirmation of life. I see the importance of accepting death in a non-fearful way and the importance of finding joy in life. For the present I continue to live in a complex world with an uncertain future, the same as everyone else.

2

History, Treatment, Prevention

A fellow cancer patient once described to me his first visit to the cancer treatment centre: "When I walked through the doorway with the word 'cancer' above it, my heart sank as the full reality of my situation hit me. I knew I was now entering a new world." Although not always the case, the common initial feeling recalls Dante's words written above the gate of hell, "Abandon hope all ye who enter here."

Cancer can occur in almost any part of the body. Often it develops in places such as the rectum, breast, prostate or cervix: areas that we feel embarrassed to talk about. It is usually silent and invisible in the early stages, but the final stages can be brutally apparent. Much money has been spent on cancer research and a great deal of information accumulated, yet the facts remain grim. The overall cure rate for all cancers is approximately 30%, a figure that has not changed much in the last thirty years.

Cancer is not a new disease. The earliest descriptions of what would later be recognized as cancer are found in Egyptian medical tracts known as the "Ebers Papyrus," written about 3,500 years ago. Ancient mummies and skeletons also show evidence of cancer. In the fourth century B.C., 2,500 years ago, the disease was first named. By then Greek physicians were familiar with such cancers as those found in the breast, stomach and uterus. Using the Greek word "karkinos" which means "crab," Hippocrates chose this image because certain cancers resemble a crab with claw-like tentacles buried deep within the flesh. The word also describes pain similar to a crab's bite. Others suggest that the image conveys the disease's crab-like spread through the body. Five hundred years later in Rome in 164 A.D., the physician Galen worked on the classification of cancer. The word "tumor" was introduced in this period. It comes from the Greek "tymbos" (a sepulchral mound) and the Latin "tumere" (to swell).

The first documentation of an occupational cancer due to environmental causes was done by Percival Pott in 1775. He noted that English chimney sweeps had developed a high incidence of cancer of the scrotum and he correlated this to the prolonged exposure of their skin to coal soot. Around the turn of the nineteenth century, the French scientist Marie Francois Bichat described cancer as a tissue. Although abnormal, it still developed somewhat like other tissues of the body. The idea that the cell is the basic unit of structure evolved in the 1830s; in 1838, after observing cancerous tumors under a microscope, the German Johannes Muller stated that cancer is cellular. Even today the cellular approach remains the basis of all cancer research. It is a widely held scientific theory that cancers begin when individual cells of the body undergo certain genetic changes called mutations.

Cancer has been recognized since ancient times. It remained a rare illness until the beginning of the Industrial Revolution in the seventeenth century when the incidence of cancer slowly began to increase. In the

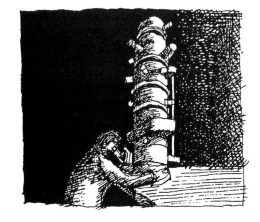

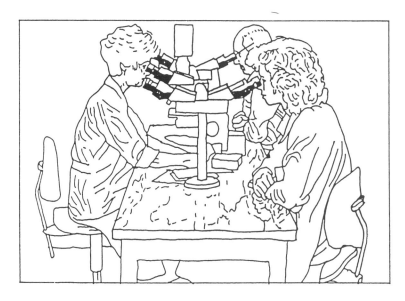

Left:
Physicians and Microscopes, 1990
Ink on paper

Below:
Child with Cancer, 1990
Ink on paper, 9.0 x 9.0 cm

Opposite:
Scientist's Vision, 1990
Ink on paper, 7.3 x 8.5 cm

early nineteenth century, Stanislas Tanchou, a French statistician, found that cancer accounted for two percent of the deaths around Paris. By the beginning of the twentieth century, the cancer rate in America had reached four percent; subsequently the situation began to change drastically. A century ago, in Canada, infectious diseases such as tuberculosis, influenza and pneumonia were the major causes of death. These infectious diseases have given way to degenerative diseases, like heart disease and cancer. Although people are living longer and thus increasing the opportunity of getting cancer, the evidence shows that even accounting for this, the cancer rate is increasing. According to the Canadian Cancer Society, one in three people will develop cancer. All ages are affected. Half of the people who die of cancer are over 65, but, alarmingly, cancer is now the most common death by disease among children.

Rates of cancer change dramatically in different regions of the world and also within regions. For

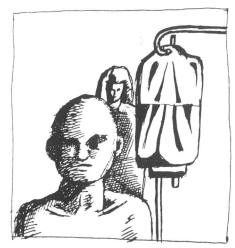

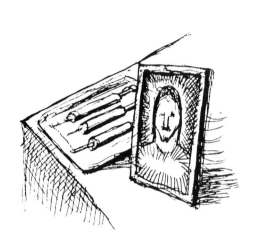

Above:
Chemotherapy and Christ, 1990
Ink on paper, 5.5 x 6.5 cm

Opposite:
Broccoli, 1991
Ink on paper, 4.0 x 6.0 cm

example, the incidence of colon cancer in the United States is ten times higher than it is in Nigeria. Information such as this has led Dr. David M. Prescott and Dr. Abraham S. Flexer to suggest in their book, *Cancer: The Misguided Cell*, that up to ninety percent of all human cancer could be prevented through changes in environment, diet and lifestyle.

Presently, the three most common treatments for cancer are surgery, radiation, and chemotherapy. Surgery is the oldest of these three. It involves cutting into the body and removing the cancerous tumor and often the surrounding tissue. Radiation was developed in the early-to-mid twentieth century. Its use consists of powerful x-rays directed at the cancer, causing it to be destroyed. Chemotherapy, or chemical therapy (treatment with drugs), was first used in the 1950s. Drugs are injected into the bloodstream and thus come in contact with the cancer cells. It has been discovered that drugs given in combination can enhance the cancer-killing effect. Over the last few decades, methods for applying these drugs have become increasingly sophisticated and subtle.

While progress has been made in treating cancers such as childhood leukemias, skin cancers, and Hodgkin's disease, the fact remains that over two-thirds of those who get cancer die within five years. However, new ideas beyond the three traditional treatments are now being explored. One new approach is immunotherapy which attempts to enhance the ability of the body's own immune system to destroy cancer cells. It involves injecting vaccines prepared from bacteria, and uses interferon, a protein produced from white blood cells. So far, results have been inconclusive and there have been no cures.

Prevention shows great promise in reducing cancer. Two methods of prevention are avoiding carcinogens and improving diet. Carcinogens are agents in our environment that cause cancer: viruses, radiation, and chemicals. In the case of the English chimney sweeps with cancer of the scrotum, coal soot was identified as the carcinogen. Their scrotal cancer was almost completely prevented simply by bathing more frequently and making sure that the chimney soot was thoroughly washed off their skin. While not all carcinogenic substances have been identified and some are in dispute or unavoidable, other agents, that can be avoided, have been clearly proven to trigger cancer. One such substance is cigarette smoke, undeniably linked to lung and other cancers. Some doctors suggest that perhaps twenty-five to thirty percent of all cancer deaths derive from tobacco.

The uncertainty of identifying carcinogens and the fact that not all people exposed to them develop cancer suggest that possibly diet may be a more fundamental means of prevention. Our diet has changed radically in the last century, mirroring the massive increase in degenerative diseases. There has been a shift away from complex carbohydrates (whole grains) towards saturated fat (meat and dairy products). Our food is also more refined (simple sugars instead of complex ones), processed, and chemicalized. Some foods are carcinogenic, such as charred meat. Other foods protect us. One study suggested that eating cabbage, Brussels sprouts, and broccoli reduced the incidence of colon and rectal cancers. Michio Kushi, a macrobiotic leader, argues that proper food can improve blood quality and strengthen the immune system, thus protecting us from cancer. The Canadian Cancer Society is now giving out nutritional information that advises people to eat more grains and vegetables and less fatty foods.

Other factors, many of which are related to lifestyle, may be connected to cancer. These include mental

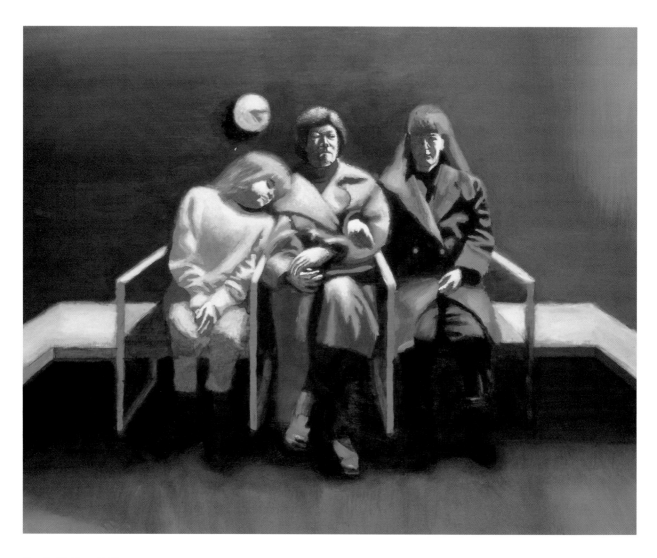

Family Waiting, 1989
Acrylic on canvas, 61.0 x 76.2 cm

attitude, exercise, and personal stress. Science is not yet able to prove that attention to and changes in these areas can help prevent cancer, but it is plainly true that having a positive frame of mind, getting regular exercise, and managing stress will make us healthier.

Many of the issues discussed in this chapter suggest cancer has its economic, political, and social consequences. Cancer has put an enormous burden on the health care system and the situation is sure to get worse as the population ages. The circumstances are so serious in my own province, Nova Scotia, that the government recently formed a commission to study this economic question. Another socio-economic aspect of cancer is its division along class lines. Those who have access to better education tend to follow healthier lifestyles, thus they are less likely to develop cancers. Even though the vast majority of cancers are preventable, most of the enormous funds spent on fighting cancer are put into treatment rather than prevention.

Industrialization, technology, and other changes in the twentieth century have dramatically altered our environment, diet, lifestyle, even our family structure. It is necessary to be aware of the consequences of these developments. Infectious diseases such as tuberculosis have declined while degenerative diseases such as heart disease and cancer have increased. As we approach the end of the twentieth century cancer is a major public health problem, affecting us both personally and socially. We need to strip away all the fantasies associated with cancer and recognize that it is a disease that can be overcome, or avoided, just as other major diseases have been. While the scientists search for a magic bullet that will cure cancer, there is still life and hope among the millions of people with cancer. Some will die, but others will continue to live fulfilling lives despite the disease, and there are others, perhaps more fortunate, who will survive the cancer completely.

3

Psychological Aspects

As I met more and more people with cancer in the hospital and in support groups I noticed that while not many were cured, not many were dying either. Some people think of cancer as a dark night they must pass through. For me, however, cancer is like an ambiguous twilight.

This element of ambiguity is heightened by our society's taboo about discussing cancer. Even today there is a language of cancer not far removed from the verbal disguises of George Orwell, a vocabulary of euphemisms such as "cyst," "tumor," "inflammation," "polyps" or "shadow."

Like AIDS, cancer is the leprosy of our age. Oddly, other major public health problems, such as heart disease, which kills more people than cancer, are not thought about in the same way. A booklet published by the Canadian Cancer Society gives an example of a woman who noticed this. While she was in the hospital for heart disease, she received amusing "Get Well" cards from her friends. But when she went in for a cancer operation, she received only sympathy cards.

The three main treatments of surgery, chemotherapy and radiation are usually effective in reducing the size of the tumor, and this relieves pain and prolongs life. Still, there is always the uncertainty that microscopic cancer cells will resist the treatment. Doctors are like technological oddsmakers, giving this woman a 30% chance of curing her ovarian cancer or that man 65% on his Hodgkin's disease.

The shifting, shadow-filled, uncertain situation of the cancer patient is contrary to a basic human need for meaning. Many people ask, "Why me?" a question that is perhaps unanswerable. Agonizing over such an issue can often lead to negative feelings of guilt and blame. Some attach moralistic overtones to certain illnesses, including cancer, seeing the sickness as a form of punishment. Others see cancer as a disease of

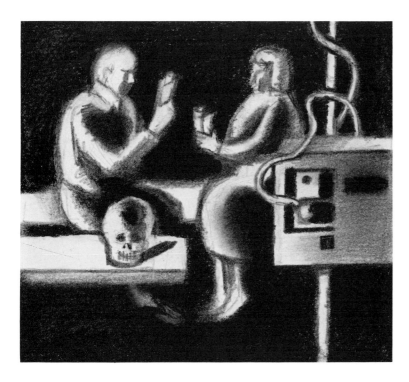

Patients Playing Cards, 1990
Charcoal on paper, 11.8 x 13.0 cm

31

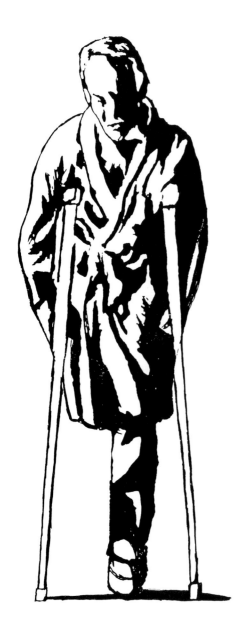

technology, affluence, and overconsumption, with uncontrolled economic growth paralleling uncontrolled tumor growth. Susan Sontag has written, "Nothing is more punitive than to give a disease a meaning, that meaning being invariably a moralistic one." She argues that the healthiest way of being ill is one that resists such thinking.

While it is wrong to attach morality to a health problem, we must also recognize that such factors as unhealthy diet and lifestyle, and a polluted environment are responsible for many of our cancers. It is important to be careful when assigning such responsibility. A physician may blame smokers for causing their lung cancers. But if that doctor, or the medical association, or society, have not spoken out against the dangers of tobacco or tried to prevent its advertising and glamourization, they are equally to blame.

How we have responded to cancer is extremely revealing of our cultural values. Present treatments reflect the anger and violence of our age. The disease is enveloped in military metaphors. We talk about the war on cancer. The illness is viewed as an enemy to be fought aggressively. Cancer cells are thought of as "invading" and "colonizing" parts of the body. The three main treatments can be related to human warfare. Surgery can be compared to hand combat with knives and swords, while chemotherapy, like the nitrogen mustard I received as part of my therapy, is synonymous with chemical weapons. Radiation could be associated with the technology of nuclear bombs. With the lack of real improvement in the five-year survival rate for most cancers, the results of the war on cancer bear disturbing similarities to futile colonial wars or our intervention in countries we do not understand.

In contrast to the medical model of war on

symptoms, there is an alternate, more wholistic, approach. From this viewpoint, symptoms are seen as friendly signs that warn of an imbalance in health, rather than enemies to be dominated. Healing is brought about by strengthening and building up the patient, and restoring health. When this happens, the symptoms will disappear. The first model emphasizes treatment and intervention; the second focuses on prevention and non-intervention.

Our society's morbid fear of death makes cancer different from other diseases. Normal relationships break down in an atmosphere of fear. A close friend has a sister-in-law with brain cancer. She confided to me, "When I go to the hospital to visit her, I just don't know what to say." People with cancer face many fears: they are frightened by lack of knowledge, they face an uncertain future, they have to deal with fear in others, but most of all, I believe, they fear being alone. It was a great help to me to be able to meet and talk with other cancer patients in the hospital. Suddenly, I was no longer isolated; sharing the experience with others somehow diminished cancer's fear-making power.

Often, however, the patients undergo a "social death" long before their actual death. Healthy people should not let their own fears about death prevent them from talking about it, thus leaving dying patients alone. Elisabeth Kübler-Ross, who has written extensively on death and dying, notes, "Dying does not have to be a nightmare unless we make one out of it."

An illness such as cancer can change us in profound ways. When I was told that my cancer had left me with a 20% chance of living, I began to evaluate my life seriously for the first time. It became much easier to put away worries about trivialities and be more objective. I came to see that I had placed too much importance on work and discovered that the real value in my life came

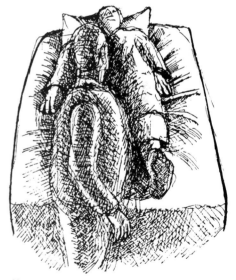

Above:
Visit, 1990
Ink on paper, 11.0 x 9.2 cm

Opposite:
Man With Amputated Leg, 1990
Ink on paper, 15.0 x 5.5 cm

33

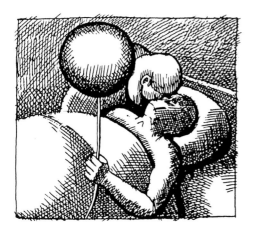

Balloon, 1990
Ink on paper, 9.5 x 10.6 cm

from relationships with family and friends. Our lives can easily become rote; we can often act like somnambulists rather than being fully alive. A disease can wake us up and make us want to enrich our lives.

I have made many friends among the cancer patients I have met, and I am continually impressed with their power to change and continue developing. One friend, of retirement age, adopted a natural foods diet, and began to feel much better. She started to serve a healthy, vegetarian meal at her restaurant, and soon she had a sizeable daily clientele, thus making a great contribution to community health. Another friend, with liver cancer, did not have long to live. I watched her complaining turn to a peaceful acceptance of death. In a touching coincidence, her daughter had a child during this time. My dying friend was able to find meaning, and happiness, in the birth of her first grandchild.

The ambiguous landscape of cancer makes for a difficult journey. The psychology is sometimes as intimidating as the actual disease. A cancer prognosis can be bleak, but as long as we are not alone there is hope. Jean Cameron, a social worker who was diagnosed ten years ago as terminally ill with cancer, writes, "When a person looks at you and loves, you are no longer ugly and unclean with disease, and each day seems a precious gift to be cherished and savoured to the full." Humans have a great capacity to adapt and to grow. In this ability rests our future in dealing with cancer, and indeed, all of life.

Images

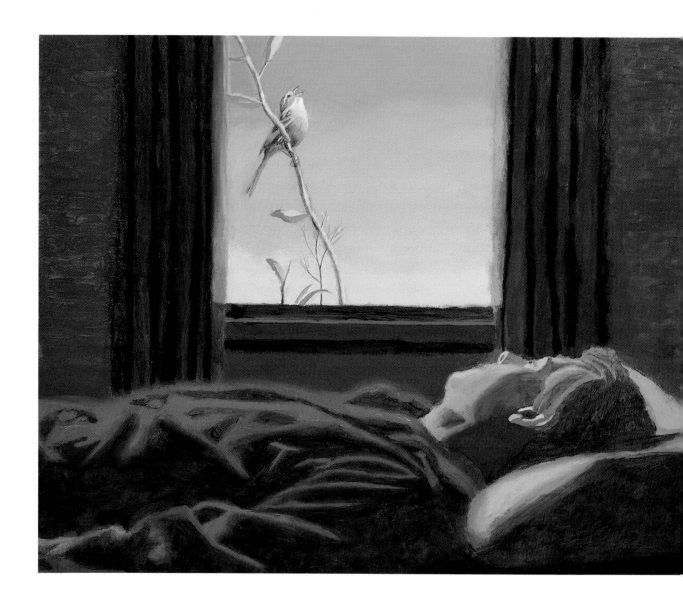

Sparrow

One haunting memory of my illness is spring in Toronto. I had gone to the Princess Margaret Hospital to receive radiation treatments. From my window in the lodge all I could see were the tops of horse-chestnut trees, covered with beautiful white blossoms. These blossoms seemed to say to me all I was feeling. They became for me encouragement to persevere, a symbol of recovery.

This image was painted three years later, with the sparrow replacing the blossoms. I have tried to contrast a number of opposites: outside and inside, the horizontal man with the vertical bird and trees, passiveness and activity, illness and health. I see the man and sparrow as equivalents. The sparrow of the title applies as much to the man as to the bird. To me, they share the same vulnerability and strength.

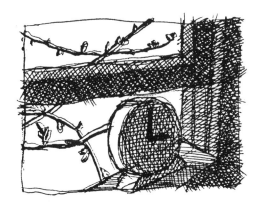

Above:
Clock in Window, 1989
Ink on paper, 5.0 x 6.5 cm

Opposite:
Sparrow, 1989
Acrylic on canvas, 61.0 x 76.2 cm

Chest X-ray

For most patients in the hospital, getting a chest x-ray is a common experience. In my case, the doctors could see and feel the cancer in my neck, and the purpose of the x-ray was to determine if the disease had spread to my chest.

On the left of the drawing is the barrel of the machine which, like a gun, directs the x-ray beam at the patient. The box on the right touching the patient's side contains the film to be exposed to the x-ray. The woman grips a bar above her head so her arms will not be part of the image. In the center of the drawing the technician is isolated in a protective booth.

The details of this rather minimal drawing have been filtered through my memory, leaving only the strongest impressions. I recall a long wait. The room was slightly cool, and dimly lit, with a feeling of technological sterility about it. For some reason I remember a sink in the corner.

It is a strange paradox of modern medicine that the useful diagnostic tool is also harmful, and the operator is shielded while the patient is not. There is an alien, bloodless, faintly eerie quality to this and other tests. It seems an absurd anomaly to be spending periods of time alone in darkened rooms filled with machines.

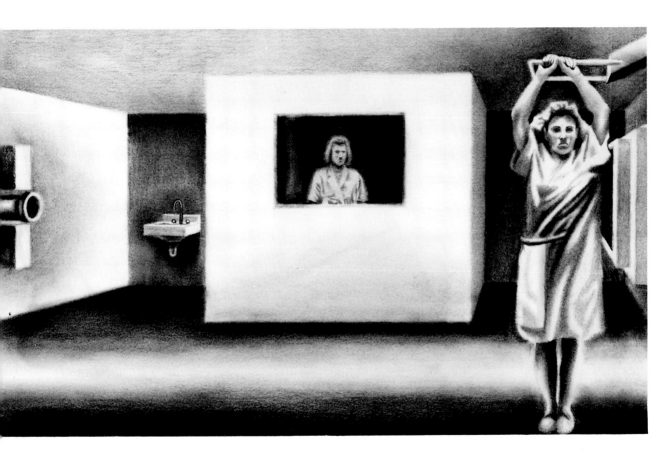

Chest x-ray, 1990
Charcoal on paper, 24.7 x 40.4 cm

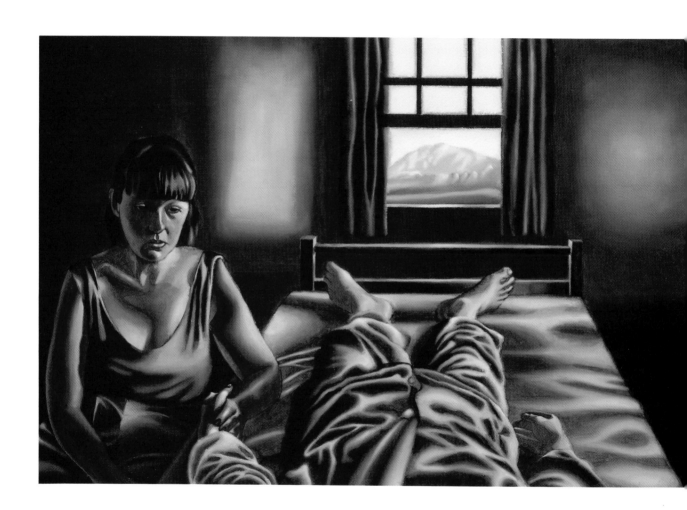

Mountain

The starting point for this painting was a song by Elvis Presley, "Lord, You Gave Me a Mountain This Time." I had already done a series of drawings using a mountain both as a metaphor for a heavy burden and as a parallel to a growing tumor. This bedroom scene, however, is primarily a relationship picture exploring human feelings under the pressure of cancer. It is a moody, atmospheric work, perhaps evoking the sense of soulfulness of country music.

Despite its central placement, the mountain is a minor element of this image. As I worked on this painting, the gesture of the figures holding hands became more important. The woman in the picture is under a great strain, her face full of mixed emotions. While there is a monumentalizing and heroic quality here, cracks are beginning to show. There is an undercurrent of dark sexuality. I imagine the room being very hot and both people covered with sweat.

Most of the people who appear in my images are friends who agree to pose, almost like actors. Although the pictures are not portraits in the strict sense of the word, I feel because I know the person being depicted, they have a sense of authenticity that would be missing if I were to use professional models. The woman in this painting is a very close friend and, in this case at least, there are elements of portraiture here.

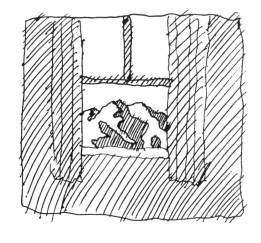

Above:
Mountain, 1990
Ink on paper, 7.0 x 8.0 cm

Opposite:
Mountain, 1990
Acrylic on canvas, 91.4 x 137.2 cm

41

Solarium

Being sick in the hospital seems to entail much waiting. Humanity is on display and, with nothing to do, we become voyeurs, looking into the intimate details of the lives of our fellow patients. While ill, I occupied some of my time by sketching other patients. Later, after I received grant money to work on this project, I again returned to hospital waiting rooms and lounges with my sketchbook.

This painting is a combination and summation of those drawings and ideas. A group of five people are shown in a hospital solarium. One man looks inward, his nose buried in a newspaper. Another man stands by a window, looking outward. The woman on the right has a third kind of look: a myoptic, catatonic gaze. In the center of the image a visiting wife embraces and kisses her husband. Above this couple, the ceiling light is like a halo.

All types of people are thrown together in these situations. There is a humiliation about being sick in public, about having life and death matters acted out in the company of strangers. As well, we are embarrassed as we are forced to confront illness in others. On the other hand, a healthy camaraderie often develops among patients. Although I did see pathetic, disturbing sights in these waiting rooms, I also saw examples of dignity and caring, which I have attempted to record in this picture.

Opposite:
Solarium, 1989
Acrylic on canvas, 61.0 x 76.2 cm

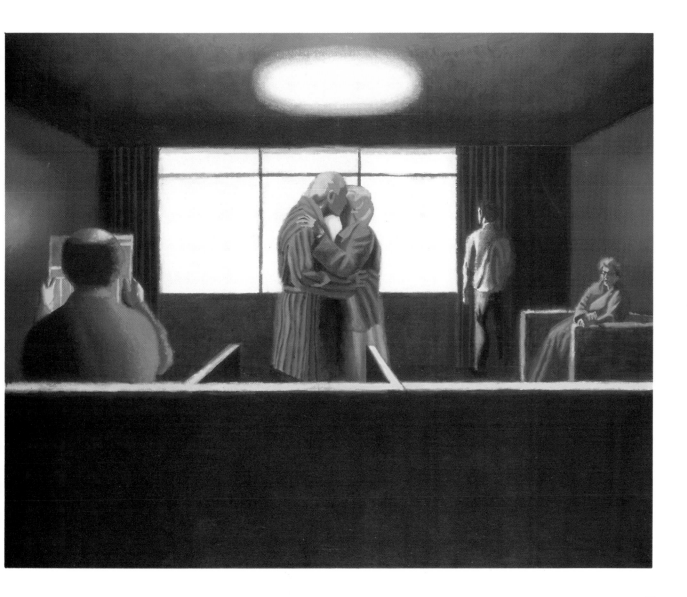

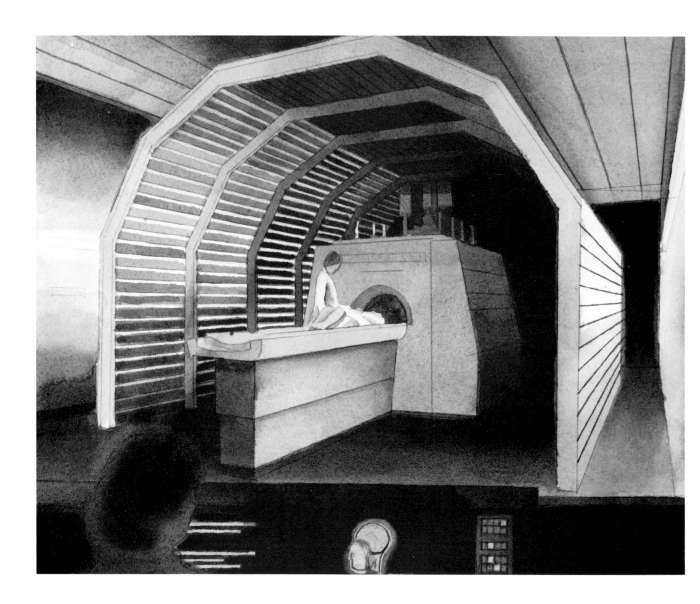

Magnetic Resonance Imager

The magnetic resonance imager, or MRI, costing two million dollars, is a high-tech machine that can see inside the human body. It uses magnetism to create its images. This watercolour shows a patient lying on a table which is being placed inside the machine by a technician. In an arc around them is a gigantic magnet, so powerful that a separate building had to be constructed to house it. The magnetism is so strong that it will destroy any watch being worn near it.

The MRI eliminates the need for certain types of diagnostic surgery. Because it works by magnetism, it avoids the potentially dangerous radiation of an x-ray. Also, unlike an x-ray, it can see through bone, making it especially useful for looking at the brain.

Technology such as this, particularly on the scale of the chapel-like MRI, evokes a sense of awe. One wonders where the end game of modern medicine will lead us. It is interesting to me, as an artist, to take note of the imagery of contemporary science. As I worked on this picture, I began to compare the magnetic resonance imager to cave paintings made in the Dordogne region of France over 30,000 years ago and noticed many similarities. Both images are produced in cave-like structures and create an atmosphere of wonder. They perform helpful functions to their respective societies and embody some of our deepest beliefs.

Opposite:
Magnetic Resonance Imager, 1989
Acrylic on paper, 25.0 x 34.0 cm

Chemotherapy

The story of cancer, like the story of any modern disease, is largely also the story of drugs. Society's attitude towards drugs is curiously ambiguous. On a physical level, they can help us while at the same time hurting us. On a social level, the same drug that is acceptable in a medical setting is not acceptable on the street, even though the drug is being used in both cases to relieve pain.

When my chemotherapy first started, I would come into the cancer clinic as an outpatient, get an injection of drugs in my arm and then go home. Eventually, the side effects became so severe that I would be checked into a bed in the hospital to get my injection and remain for a few days afterward. The nurse would prepare the syringes, bring them into my room and set them on the bedside table. The moments waiting for the doctor to perform the injection were even more difficult psychologically than the taxing physical reactions to follow. The brutality of chemotherapy made me feel very cowardly as the nurse held my hand and told me how much it would help me.

Chemotherapy is a psychological painting about drugs. The chemical in the syringe is Adriamycin which I received in combination with three other drugs. A woman in her eighties, with lymphatic cancer, who was getting chemotherapy, posed for this picture. She is wearing a turban because the treatments have caused her hair to fall out. I have attempted to evoke the mixture of good and bad feelings triggered by the patient's thoughts about the drug. The chemical lies in the syringe, red like the color of life or the color of alarm. The encounter between human and drug, an all-too-telling twentieth century relationship, is played out here.

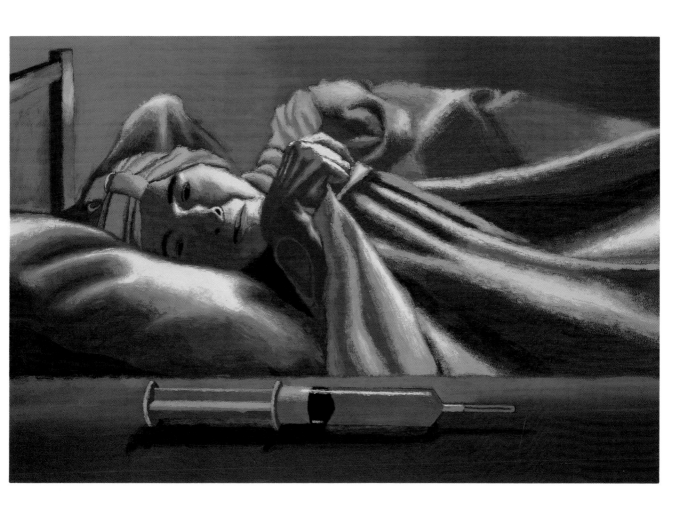

Chemotherapy, 1989
Acrylic on canvas, 61.0 x 91.4 cm

Family Illness

This painting was done quite early on in the project, and it is a picture about family relationships. The woman who posed in bed is a friend who actually had cancer. The others are her daughter and friend, who are both involved in acting.

A disease such as cancer cannot help but affect members of the patient's family. This image focuses on the relationship between the two young people, who could be brother and sister, or husband and wife. The symmetrical composition places the cancer patient, symbolically and physically, at the center of the family, dividing it in two.

The look between the man and woman is highly charged with psychological and emotional tension, communicating volumes, and nothing at all. On the patient's left is one form of maintenance, an intravenous (IV) bag. On her right is another means of sustenance, a can of pop, placed beside a clock. The cancer patient lies in bed like a ghost with the mental fireworks of the others imploding in the silence around her.

Opposite:
Family Illness, 1989
Acrylic on canvas, 76.2 x 101.6 cm

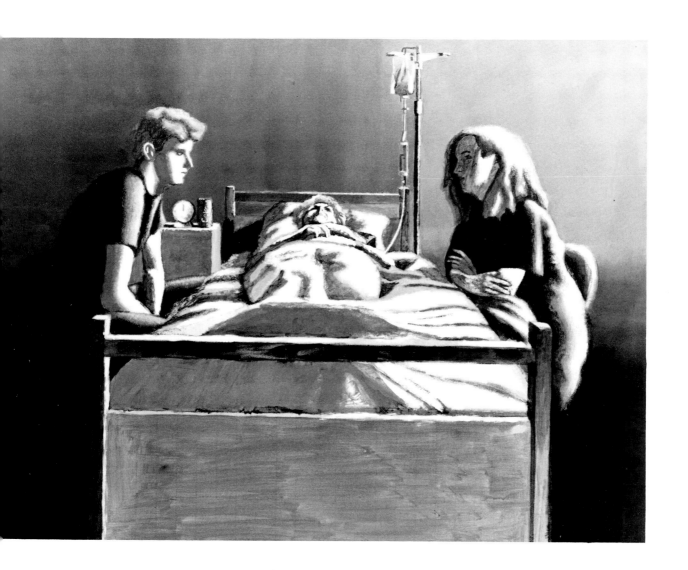

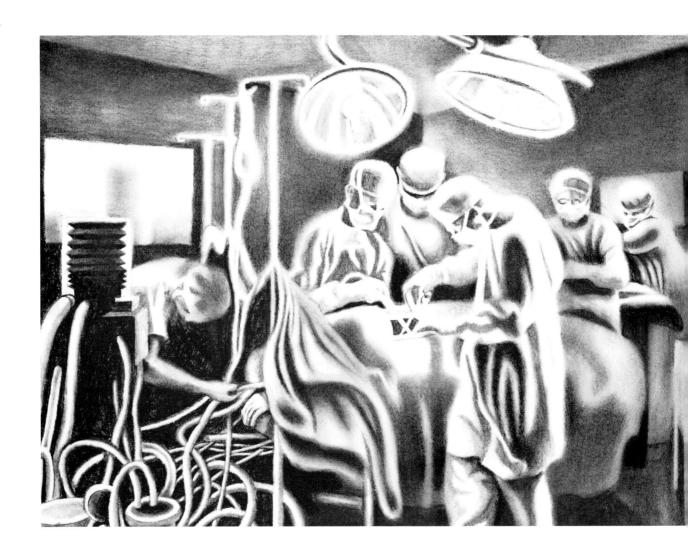

Lung Operation

My memories of my two biopsies are rather indistinct as
I was given preparatory drugs before each operation. I
vaguely remember an early morning, a lot of bustle
around me, feeling cold under the sheet, then the
anesthetist above me, then nothing, then feeling fuzzy,
and finally feeling sore.

Surgery is perhaps the most mechanical form of
medicine. Patients are wheeled in to have parts
removed, replaced or repaired. One of the anesthetists
felt that there was a different atmosphere here in
comparison to other medical areas. Because the patient
is not conscious, there is a more relaxed, casual feeling,
almost like in a garage. I noticed a radio softly played in
the corner of the operating room.

One surgeon discussed with me the nature of his
work. He deals primarily with lung cancer, and most of
the patients he gets are cases without much hope. In
fact, he is able to cure only about 10% of those he
operates on. With the others it is a matter of
temporarily relieving discomfort, and prolonging life for
a year or two.

This drawing shows a typical surgical team. On the
left, by a respirator, amid a jumble of tubes coming in
and going out of the patient, is the anesthetist. In the
centre are three physicians: senior surgeon, resident
and intern. On the right is the head nurse and a scrub
nurse. The patient lies under a sheet. The doctors have
cut into his side and are removing part of his lung. They
stand under bright lights, skilled human mechanics, at
work in the city.

Opposite:
Lung Operation, 1991
Charcoal on paper, 29.6 x 40.4 cm

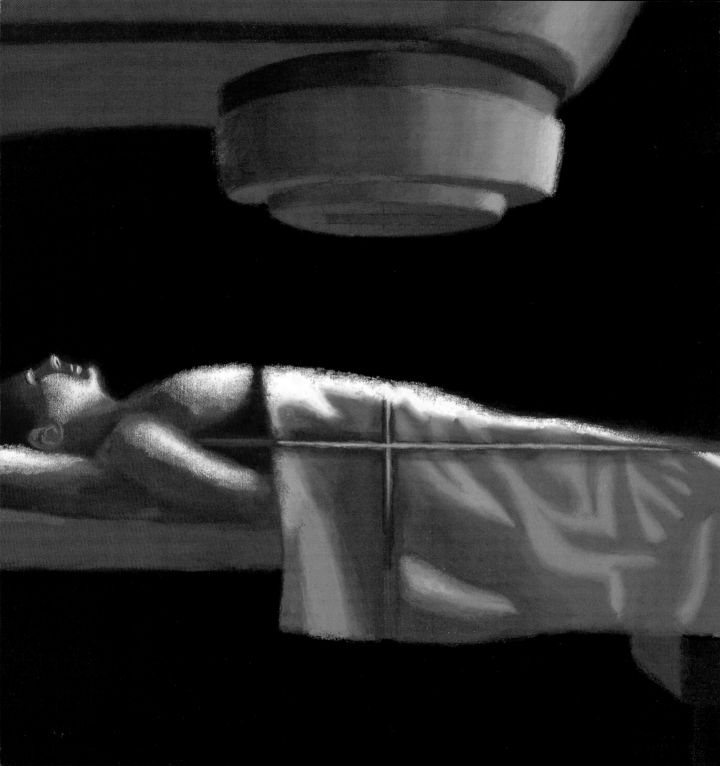

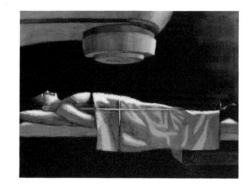

Radiation

Of the three main treatments for cancer, radiation is the "cleanest." In surgery, the body is cut into with a knife. In chemotherapy, the body is pierced with a needle or a pill is taken. Radiation, in contrast, is invisible. Like an x-ray, it renders the body transparent.

This image depicts a man lying underneath a radiation machine. The rays of radiation are directed at his abdominal area. There are allusions to religious rituals in this picture: the red lasers which are used for positioning suggest a Christian cross, the table the man lies on is like an altar, he is covered with a white shroud, the machine hovers above him like an idol or faceless god that must be propitiated with bodily sacrifices.

I underwent about a month of treatments very similar to those shown here. It is a strange feeling to be alone in a room lying under one of those machines, a bit like a 1950s science fiction movie. However clinical and unreal it may seem, the effects of radiation are real enough. It is equally effective in killing healthy cells as cancerous ones.

Above:
Radiation, 1989
Acrylic on canvas, 76.2 x 101.6 cm

Opposite:
Radiation (detail)

53

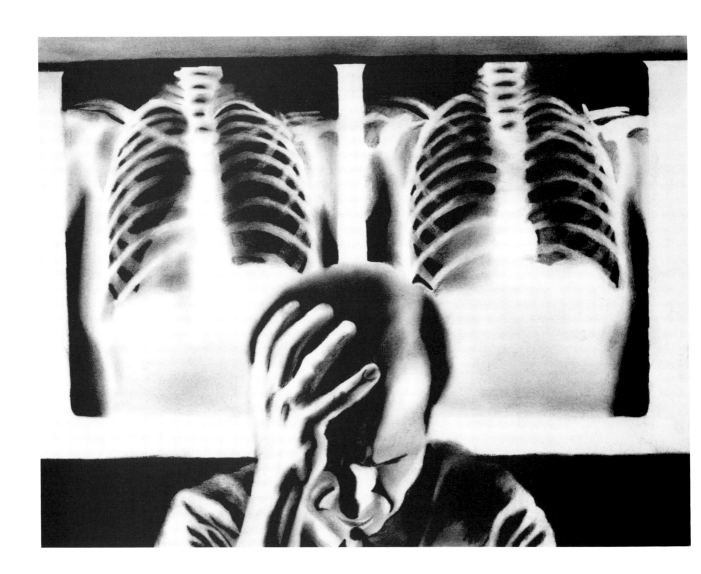

54

Doctor and X-rays

Many cancers are not apparent to the human eye.
Cancerous tumors may develop around organs deep
within the body. The x-ray is an extremely effective way
of seeing inside the body in order to study what is going
on. A doctor can examine x-rays taken of the same
patient at different times and know exactly how much
the tumor has increased. The paradox with cancer is
that this amazing ability to see through flesh is offset by
our failure to understand the cause or cure in most
cases.

In this drawing, mind and body come together. The
two chest x-rays glow iconically on the viewing screen
like crucified skeletons. The doctor holds his head in
frustration. He can see, God-like, into the patient's
chest but he cannot understand, human-like, what is
happening.

Opposite:
Doctor and X-rays, 1990
Charcoal on paper, 30.5 x 40.0 cm

Mother and Son

Family support is one of the major factors in healing, just as family conflict can often be a contributing factor in becoming ill. I know of very few cancer patients who do well without active family involvement. From this perspective, when the individual has cancer, the family has cancer.

My mother, Isabel, lent me particularly strong support during an especially difficult series of radiation treatments at the Princess Margaret Hospital in Toronto. This watercolour is based on a sketch I made while lying in bed at the hospital. I was in bad shape at this time. I could hardly hold the pencil, I felt nauseous, and I could barely see.

I have since done a number of versions of this image, but I like this watercolour best. It is crude and cartoon-like, but also a direct and heartfelt tribute.

This page:
Mother and Son, 1989
Ink on paper, 34.0 x 42.0 cm

Opposite:
Mother and Son, 1989
Acrylic on paper, 25.0 x 34.0 cm

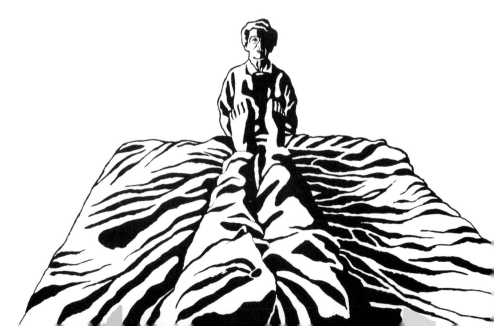

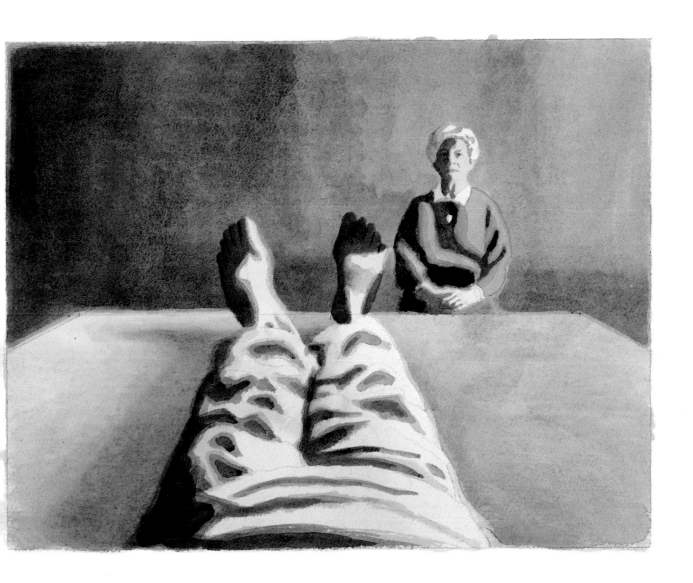

Self-Portrait with Dr. Langley

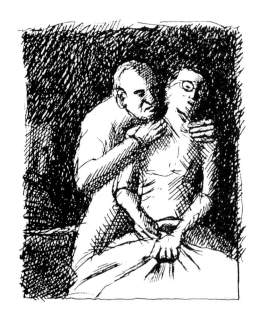

Above:
Self-portrait with Dr. Langley, 1990
Ink on paper, 10.8 x 8.8 cm

Opposite:
Self-Portrait with Dr. Langley, 1990
Charcoal on paper, 40.6 x 33.4 cm

One of my approaches to this project has been the employment of my own memories as a source of imagery. The initial symptom of my cancer, Hodgkin's Disease, was enlargement of lymph nodes in my neck. In all medical examinations I get, this is the first thing that is checked, and that is what this picture shows. Dr. Ross Langley has been overseeing treatment of my cancer since 1982. This drawing examines my relationship with him, and issues in doctor/patient relationships in general.

The relationship between doctor and patient is a special one. It recalls that between parent and child or priest and layperson, in two ways: first the doctor, like parent or priest, has more power, more knowledge; second, there is the intimacy and privacy of a family or confessional. This is contrasted with the professional, scientific neutrality of most medical settings. It is further emphasized as the patient takes off his or her clothes while the doctor is fully dressed. In my case, our ages are such that Dr. Langley could be my father.

One patient, with terminal lung cancer, compared going for a C-T scat to facing a judgement. He recalled, "I knew the verdict would be bad, it was just a question of how bad." I have tried to show on my face here the psychological tension caused by the question, "Has the cancer recurred?"

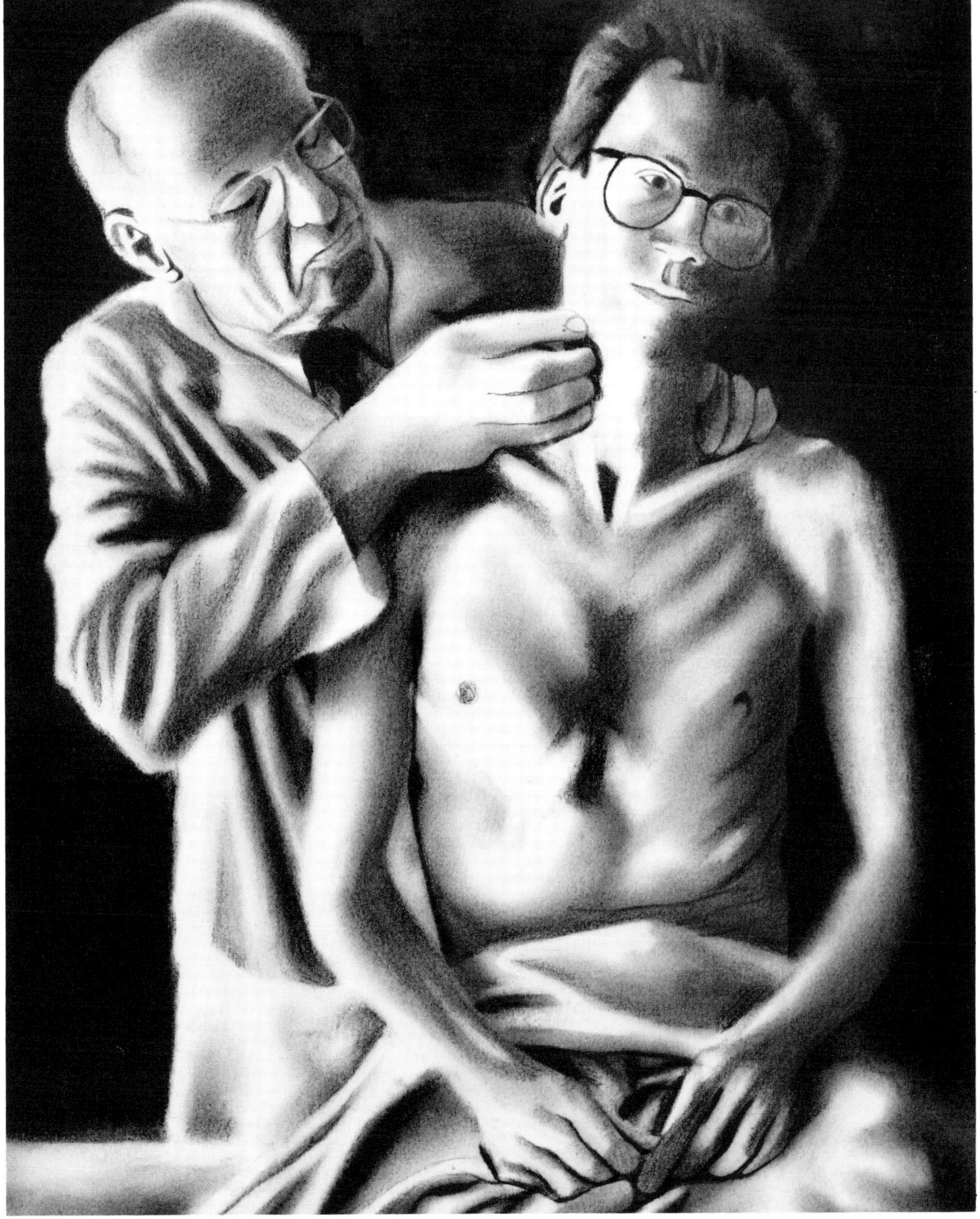

Food

Opposite:
Food, 1990
Acrylic on canvas, 97.8 x 121.9 cm

I spent over a month working every day on this large painting in which the overriding theme is food. The slice of pie at the bottom center sets the tone for the interrelationships that occur within the picture, all of which can be seen in the context of nurturing. While the sick woman is physically fed by her husband, she also receives nourishment from her relationship to her family, from the man on the television screen, from the IV solution and even from the city outside her window.

Each of these things affects the patient, though they may not all be healthy, and may even work at cross-purposes to each other. This is a familiar scene to those who spend a lot of time in hospitals. Here, under the high-key colors and the pie-in-the-sky hopes of the contemporary world, I have tried to create an image of family survival.

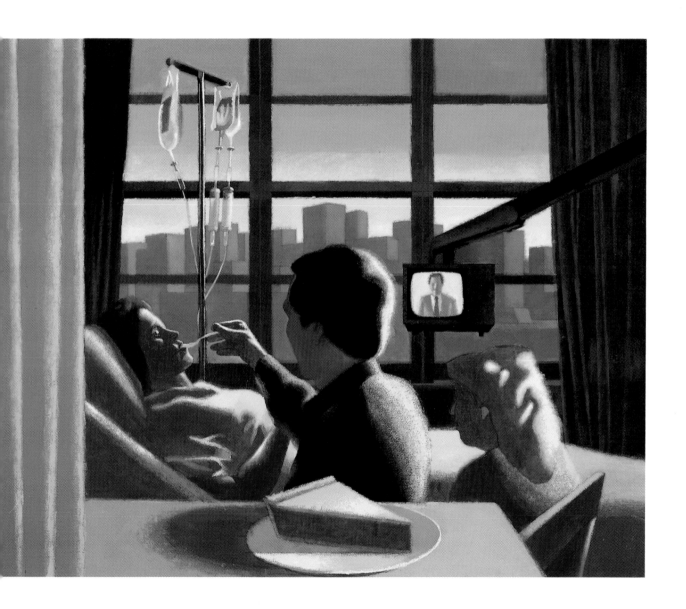

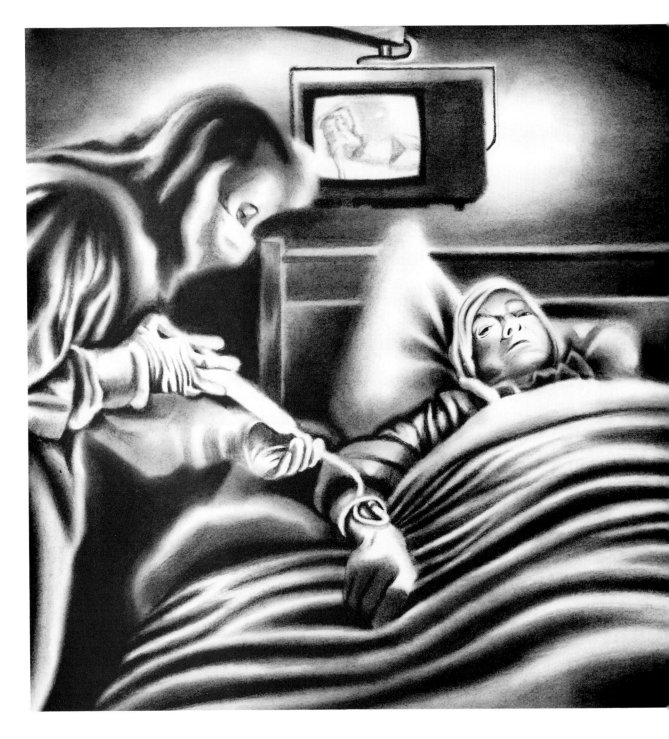

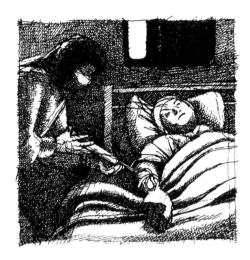

Chemotherapy Injection

Chemotherapy is given in many ways: administered by pills, injected by syringe as shown here, or dripped from an IV bag. The most usual method today is to implant surgically a device called a port-a-cath, connected to a main artery in the patient's chest, through which the chemotherapy is mechanically pumped from an IV bag Chemotherapy can be received at home, in an outpatient clinic, or in the hospital. It is very expensive; the drugs for an average treatment cost approximately $450.

The chemotherapy I received twice a month was very similar to that being given to the woman in this drawing. Side effects vary widely, depending on the patient. Injection days were the worst days of my life. Like me, the woman pictured here winces as the treatment is administered. The mindlessness of the TV playing in the background was a welcome, if unsuccessful, relief. The gap between the fantasy images on television and the reality of cancer treatment became cruelly apparent.

Above:
Chemotherapy Injection, 1990
Ink on paper, 11.6 x 12.0 cm

Opposite:
Chemotherapy Injection, 1990
Charcoal on paper, 35.6 x 35.6 cm

63

Visitors

As I began to heal, my art began to change. The fragmented views of isolated individuals and couples began to shift to a more wholistic social vision. I began to include more people within the frame of the picture.

This painting is like a psychological ecosystem, where the worlds of healthy and sick meet. The patient is seen in the context of his community. The focus is on the response of the patient's community which is both positive and negative. The emotions are varied, ranging from concern to indifference, from pessimism to support. Many of the people are brightly painted, like flowers.

The image is framed by two opposing forces. On the right, the man aggressively gesturing downward can be interpreted as having a negative meaning. The gift of a book from the woman on the left can be seen as a positive gesture and, ultimately, a symbol of hope.

There are autobiographical aspects to this painting, as most of the models were drawn from my own family and friends. The mood may be somber, but I feel this is an optimistic work, expressing faith in the continuity of our human community.

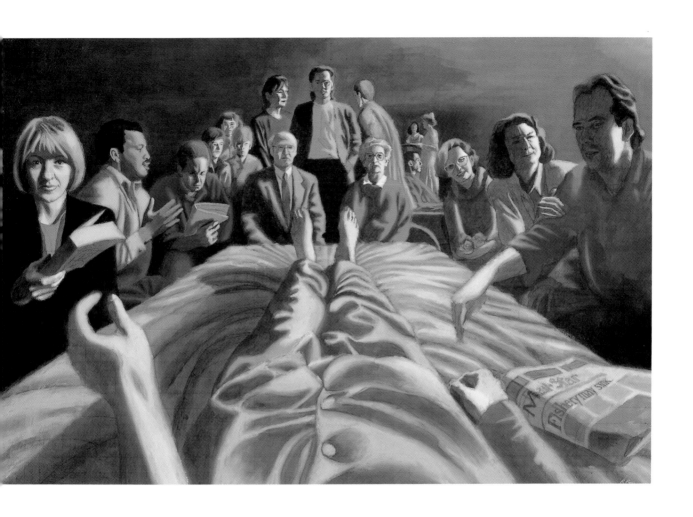

Visitors, 1989
Acrylic on canvas, 81.3 x 121.9 cm

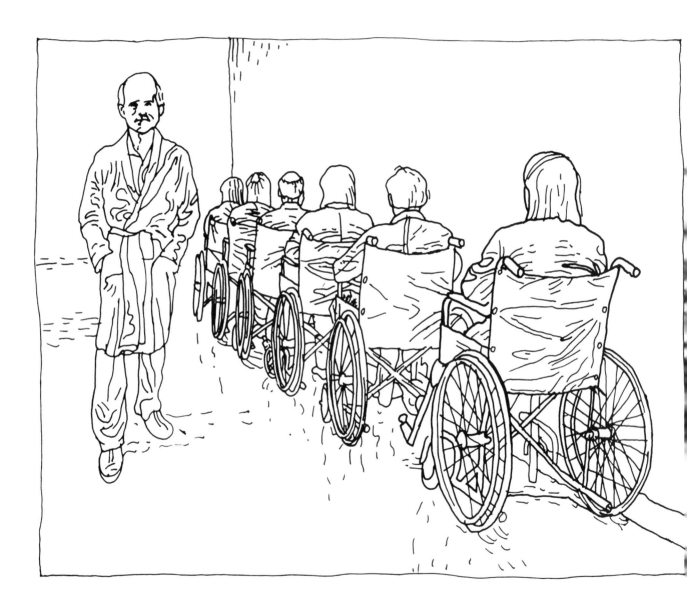

Wheelchairs

Life in the hospital reflects life on the outside. The development of the public hospital is part of the process of industrialization. Hospitals are "healing factories." The human body is a machine that has broken down and needs to be serviced by trained health mechanics.

Patients experience the same bureaucracy and line-ups as healthy people. I had to wait in line for everything: to be admitted into the hospital, for tests, for treatment, even to see the doctor after I was released.

This drawing is based on actual observation. Patients who are to have x-rays are brought from various areas of the hospital in wheelchairs and wait in the corridor for their turn. As I sat in this line-up I felt as though I were on an assembly line. On the left of the picture a man walks in the opposite direction. He has been "cured" and he rolls off the assembly line as good as new.

Opposite:
Wheelchairs, 1989
Ink on paper, 19.3 x 24.0 cm

View from Above

In my art I like to work in series. This gives the opportunity to explore one subject in depth, to examine it from many angles. A visual parallel to this search for depth in content is to portray the motif from several points of view.

Numerous images in this body of work depict a sick person in bed with various figures gathered around. I have chosen viewpoints from the foot, the sides, and the head of the bed. In this charcoal drawing, done of a real patient in Toronto's Princess Margaret Hospital, I have chosen a vantage point above the bed. The viewer's eye is close to the IV bag, the cord of which spirals down into the bedridden woman's chest. At the foot of the bed is a doll, smiling obliviously, and at the side are a man and woman.

When we see something often enough, we develop a category of blindness. Here, perhaps the unusual angle of depiction can be a means to think about what is shown in a new way.

Opposite:
View from Above, 1990
Charcoal on paper, 33.6 x 33.6 cm

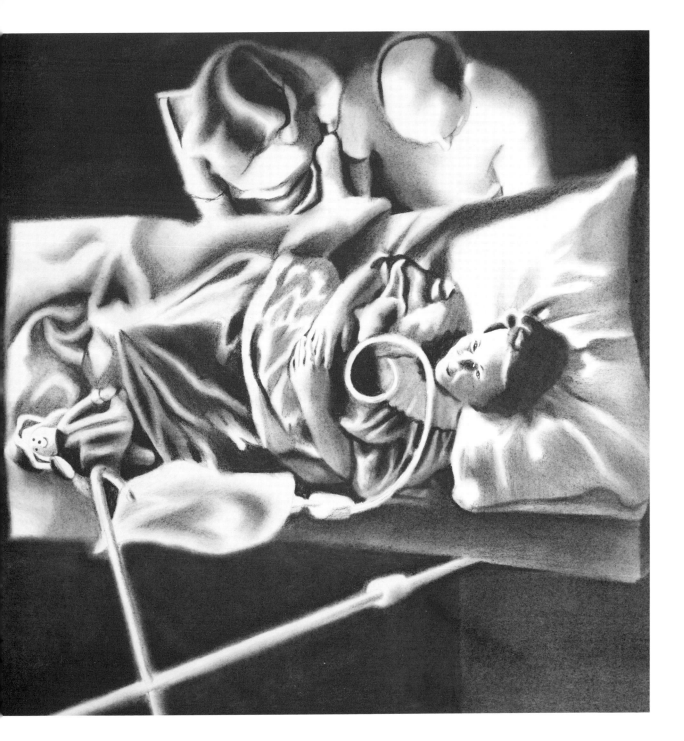

Chemotherapy and Christ

This drawing about drugs and religion had its beginnings in a photograph by Mal Warshaw showing a woman in bed with a picture of Jesus Christ on the table beside her. I began to think about Marx's quote about religion being the opium of the people. To explicitly connect these I added a tray of syringes beside the picture of Christ.

    In our age, even though people may not admit it, liberal humanism, with faith in science, has replaced faith in religion. Robert Mendelsohn, M.D. has written, "But drugs aren't merely scientific — they're sacred. Like the communion wafer which Catholics receive on the tongue, drugs are the communion wafers of Modern Medicine. When you take a drug, you're communing with one of the mysteries of the Church: the fact that the doctor can alter your inward and outward state if you have the faith to take the drug."

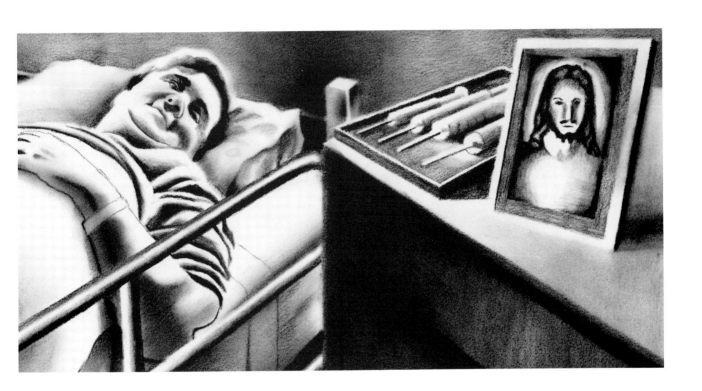

Chemotherapy and Christ, 1990
Charcoal on paper, 20.8 x 40.4 cm

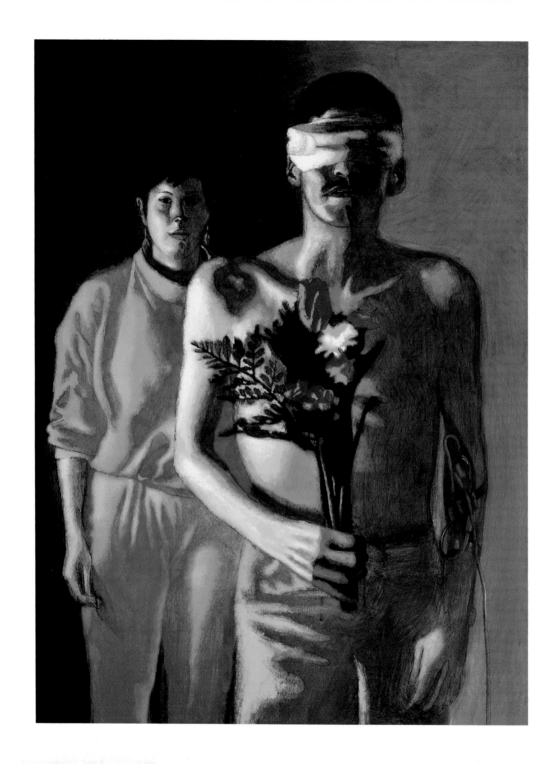

Cancer

This idea started as a depiction of an overcrowded hospital ward. There was a man in the foreground with bandaged eyes standing beside some card players. In the background were doctors, nurses, other patients, a janitor, a technician carrying a tray of syringes, and a distant figure in a doorway. I later added an embracing couple, a television, and flowers.

In this version, I kept eliminating elements until I was left with what I was most interested in: the interior journey of the man and the psychological relationship between him and his wife. The figure of the man integrates symbols of life (the flowers) and death (blindness). The bandage over the man's eyes reflects the unknown that he, and we all, encounter when we face death. This quality of the unknown is one of the most frightening aspects of having cancer. Again, the play of opposites creates tension in this work. A dialogue is set up between woman/man, clothed/unclothed, sight/blindness, and healthy/sick.

Right:
Cancer, 1990
Ink on paper, 13.2 x 6.5 cm

Left:
Cancer, 1990
Acrylic on canvas, 101.6 x 76.2 cm

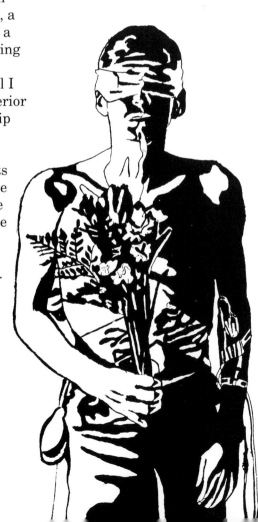

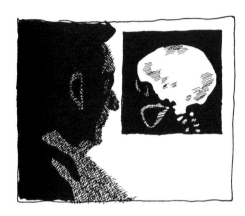

Above:
Solid and Transparent Man, 1989
Ink on paper, 8.3 x 10.1 cm

Opposite:
X-ray Viewing Room, 1990
Charcoal on paper, 28.6 x 43.2 cm

X-ray Viewing Room

Friends have commented that this image looks as if it could be a scene from *Star Trek*. The subject of this charcoal drawing is, however, the room where physicians can view and examine x-rays. There are light boxes on all the walls, and many x-ray photographs can be inspected at once.

Like other areas of the x-ray department, this room has a ghostly, surreal quality. It is darkened, and the x-ray pictures, showing sections of the body in negative, float on the screen. The light bounces crazily off the metal, plastic, and tiled surfaces.

The main reason, I believe, for this ghostly feeling is the lack of any flesh-and-blood presence of the patient. The x-ray images fragment and reverse the human body. Mrs. Smith becomes a piece of film showing a two-centimeter shadow on the lung.

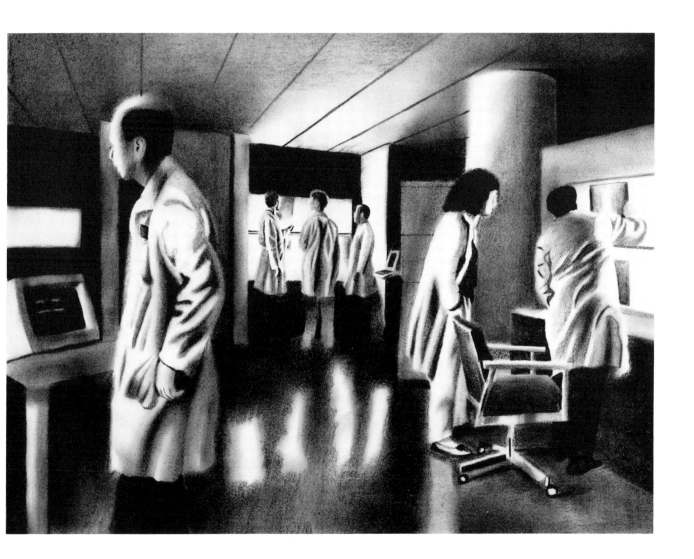

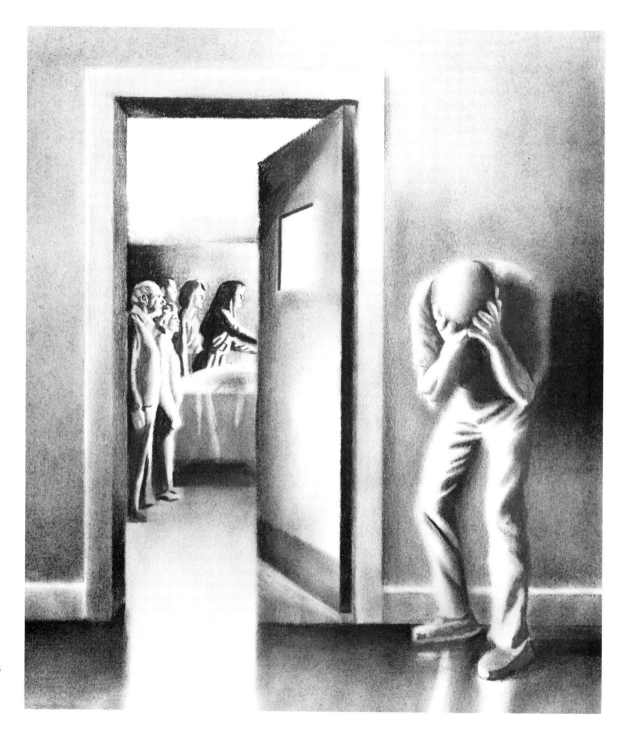

A Friend's Story

Over the course of my work in making images of cancer I have talked to and interviewed many dozens of cancer patients and their families. This image of public and private pain came out of a conversation with a friend. It is based on her description:

> Last year, my 41-year-old sister-in-law was diagnosed as having a malignant brain tumor. All members of my immediate large family flew home to Cape Breton from wherever they were living at the time — in my case, Toronto. I clearly remember the initial scene as everyone gathered around Donna's hospital bed. It had been a long time since we had all been in the same room together. Nobody knew what to say, either to Donna or to each other; in our collective state of shock, none of us knew what the appropriate reaction should be. So, in effect, we made it up as we went along.

She described to me how not everyone could fit inside the hospital room and how some of the family would have to wait in the hall. It was here, out of sight of the patient, that family members could allow their grief to be fully expressed.

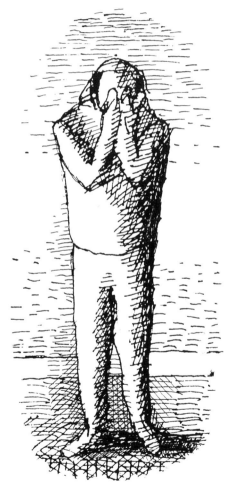

Right:
Relative, 1990
Ink on paper, 8.0 x 3.0 cm

Left:
A Friend's Story, 1990
Charcoal on paper, 36.4 x 31.6 cm

Elevator

Every time I am in the hospital elevator now, I feel I am in this painting. There seem to be more people there each time I visit. Indeed, as the population ages, and more children develop cancer, the numbers of patients coming to the cancer clinic is truly increasing. I chose to paint an elevator packed with people to convey an impression of overcrowded, overflowing claustrophobia.

A painter friend, Sue Rogers, wrote to me, "I haven't been able to shake the impact your paintings had on me this summer. In *Elevator* the faces stare out at the viewer in an imploring way, there is a feeling of otherworldliness."

In a sense, these people are phantoms. In the eyes of the world, a cancer diagnosis is a symbolic death sentence. To further this apparition-like quality, I depicted the architecture with a Kafkaesque vagueness, and handled the lighting using a dim, flickering chariscuro, overrun by deep shadows.

Here are young, old, different races, health care workers, and patients. On the right is Terry Fox, Canada's most public cancer victim. The bursting elevator transports them, like Charon's ferry, through a Homeric underworld, a dark place filled with shadows.

Opposite:
Elevator, 1989
Acrylic on canvas, 104.1 x 76.2 cm

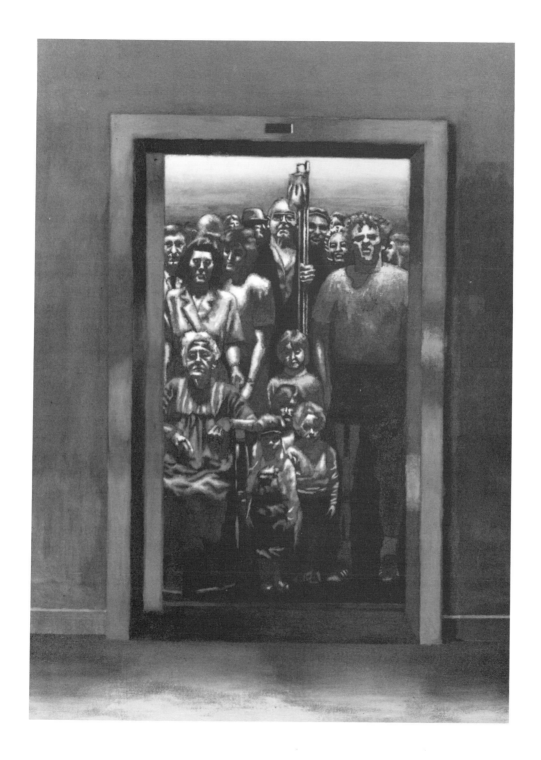

Erica

Nineteenth century artists and writers tended to romanticize tuberculosis, a major illness of the day. Young people, especially, were described as becoming more beautiful as they became flushed with the disease. Unlike tuberculosis, cancer is resistant to romantic metaphors. It just seems brutal, ugly and mean. Cancer in older people carries with it a tacit acknowledgement of inevitability, but in children we are surprised, and uncomprehending.

I spent an afternoon in the children's hospital in Halifax with a young mother and her daughter Erica. They were from Glace Bay, 300 miles away, and were both staying at the hospital while Erica received chemotherapy. Erica was suffering from a cold and so her treatment had been delayed for a few days. Although she was obviously feeling miserable, I found her playful and inquisitive. She seemed interested in seeing the paintings I had previously done and in posing for my camera. In this drawing, Erica, with her hair gone from the treatments, touches the pump that administers her chemotherapy. Her delicate gesture soundlessly conveys much of her predicament.

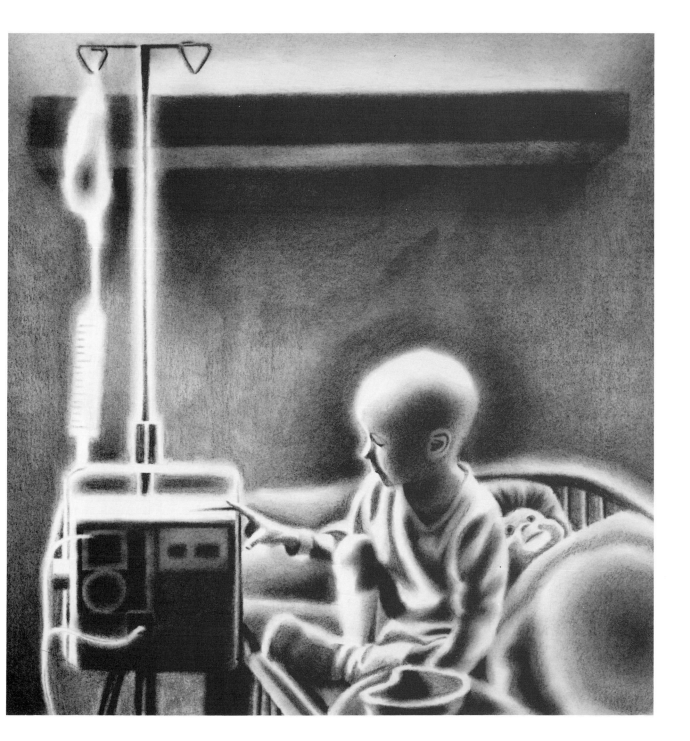

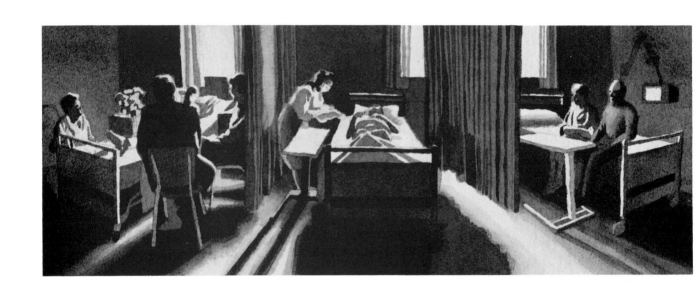

Three Beds, 1990
Acrylic on paper, 14.3 x 38.6 cm

Three Beds

Two summers ago, I read Alexander Solzhenitsyn's *Cancer Ward*, surely one of the best novels written about cancer. In it, he describes the dynamics of a cancer ward where eight men of different temperaments and backgrounds are thrown together, with only their disease in common. During my illness, I spent most of my time on the west wing of the eighth floor of Halifax's Victoria General Hospital. I was occasionally given a single or double room, but usually I shared a room with three others. I found it a little unnerving to be sharing close quarters with men I did not know, but because we were fellow-expatriates from the world of the healthy, a bond of sorts did develop.

In my paintings, I like to compare and contrast things, fashioning a visual dialectic. In *Three Beds*, the mini-world of a cancer ward is re-created. On the left a family visits, in the center a patient receives a needle, on the right a couple sit silently together, beyond the need or consolation of words. In a cancer ward, private matters become semi-public, with only the curtain between the beds providing a semblance of sanctum.

Vision

This image is half Charles Dickens and half Carl Jung. Like many of my paintings, it represents a dream or mental projection of the patient. The choir is a symbol of community. One positive quality of cancer, or any serious illness, is the way it causes us to focus and consider priorities, perhaps for the first time. Here, the man is awakening to the awareness of the importance of community.

The meaning of this picture is in the relationship between the individual and the group. Social isolation can often lead to the development of illness. Ironically, getting cancer can also lead to social isolation. Tension is created here by the distance between the man and the choir. It is not clear whether or not he will be able to get out of bed and join them.

I had trouble painting this picture. I completely repainted the choir three times, each time making them more distant. To draw a distinction between the two main elements, I painted the man wet-in-wet while I used impasto and dry brush techniques on the choir. Although this image is dark, with nightmarish overtones, it is tempered by the title *Vision*. This suggests the development of awareness, which is the first step towards healing.

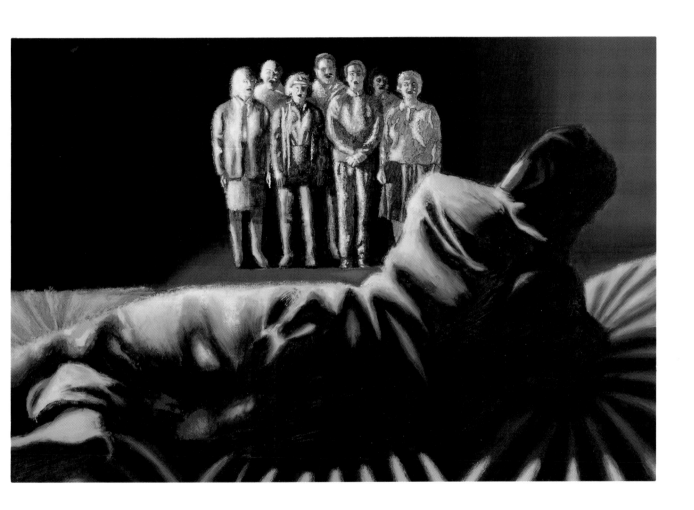

Vision, 1990
Acrylic on canvas, 81.3 x 121.9 cm

85

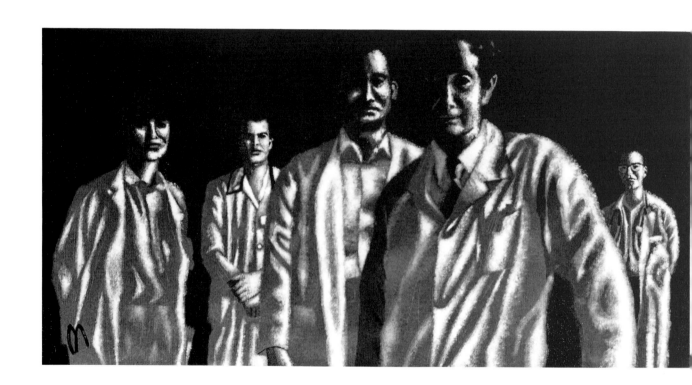

Doctors

When one doctor I know saw this painting, he was
shocked at how the physicians had been portrayed.
Here, a group of five doctors is seen from the
perspective of a patient lying in bed. Bathed in a
religious purple light, and glowing brightly against the
pitch black, some doctors loom over the patient like
giant white ghosts, others trail off, disorientingly, into
the distance. I chose an extremely coarse canvas for this
picture and the rough texture breaks up the paint into a
druggy blur. The physicians are seen as distant and
intimidating authority figures.

Today, doctors occupy a position in our society that
was once held by religious leaders. They are our secular
priests and scientific knowledge has become our
scripture. As well as being threatening, however, I have
tried to show them as individual human beings. They
sincerely want us to get better. I especially wanted to
achieve a feeling of compassion and sympathy on the
part of the nearest doctor. I see him as a kindly
television doctor in an episode that was too realistic to
be aired.

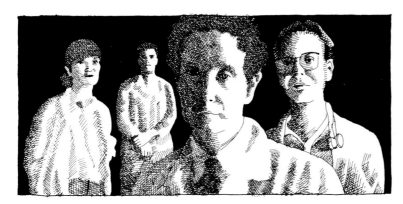

This page:
Doctors, 1990
Ink on paper, 10.7 x 23.2 cm

Opposite:
Doctors, 1990
Acrylic on canvas, 56.0 x 112.0 cm

Three Men

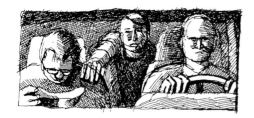

Most cancer patients receive their chemotherapy as outpatients, coming in to the clinic to get injected, and then going home. When my treatments first started, I was living in the country at my parents' home. I would usually drive into the city with my father and brother for the day. I received my treatment just before we left to drive back. I started to throw up in the car shortly after we got on the road, and I am sure this is an experience many other cancer patients share.

This image is based on these memories. I intended to show the feelings of confinement I felt during this trip, but this picture seems to have become more about what the others are thinking and feeling. The drive was difficult for me, and it must have been equally difficult for them. The psychological focus of this inky black charcoal drawing is on my father's face. The car is a cage. He is driving, but he is not in control. I was thinking of the family's journey through night in a car as a metaphor for the cancer experience, as well as a larger societal comment. We are in motion and we are trapped.

Above:
Three Men, 1990
Ink on paper, 5.2 x 11.7 cm

Opposite:
Three Men, 1990
Charcoal on paper, 32.0 x 38.0 cm

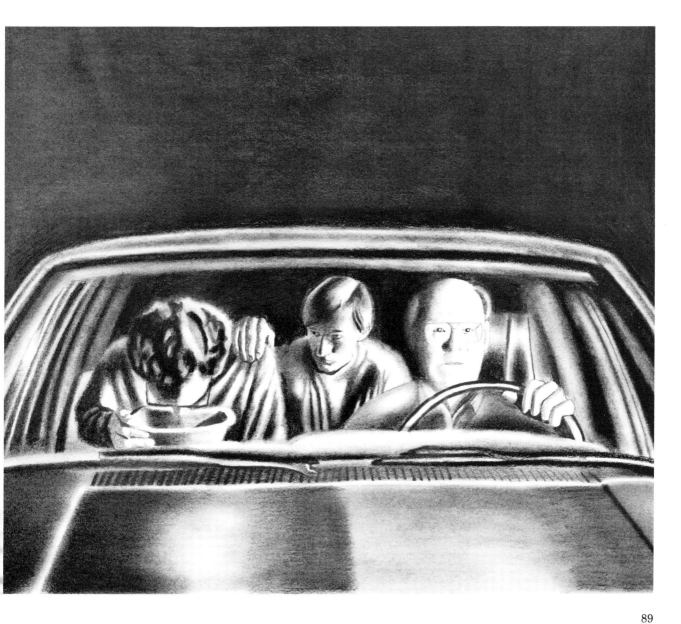

Mr. S. Is Told He Will Die

As part of my research for this project, I spent a few days following a group of doctors on their morning rounds. I put on a white coat and as far as the patient knew, I was just another doctor.

The most poignant moment came one morning when we met with a man in his sixties with liver cancer. He happened to be holding a cross as the two senior doctors sat on either side of him. Very gently, they explained to him that there was nothing further they could do for him, that he would die from his cancer, and that he could go home and be with his wife and daughters. This man had been denying his illness, but now he confronted reality for the first time. It was an incredibly intense moment, a breakthrough for the patient and doctors.

Elisabeth Kübler-Ross has named five stages of dying: denial, rage, bargaining, depression, and acceptance. The doctors handled Mr. S. with honesty and compassion, and they broke through his denial. I have tried to portray the next stages of dying that Mr. S.'s mind must have been rushing through.

In this painting, the cross symbolizes religion, and the doctors, in their white lab coats, symbolize science. The man is grasping onto both: and neither one can save his life and he knows this.

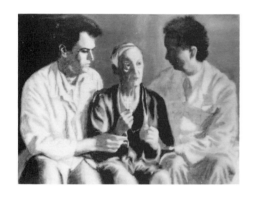

Above:
Mr. S. Is Told He Will Die, 1989
Acrylic on canvas, 76.2 x 101.6 cm

Opposite:
Mr. S. Is Told He Will Die (detail)

90

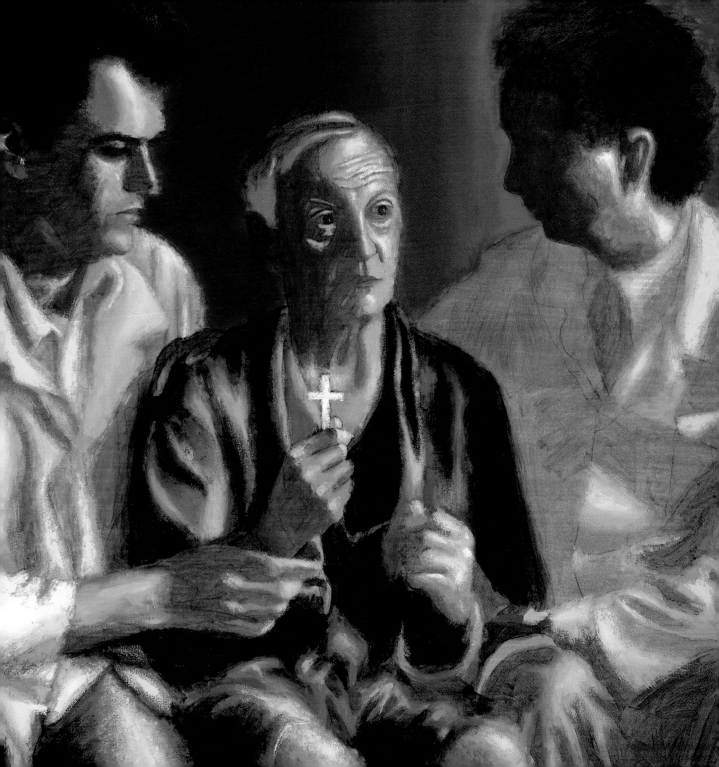

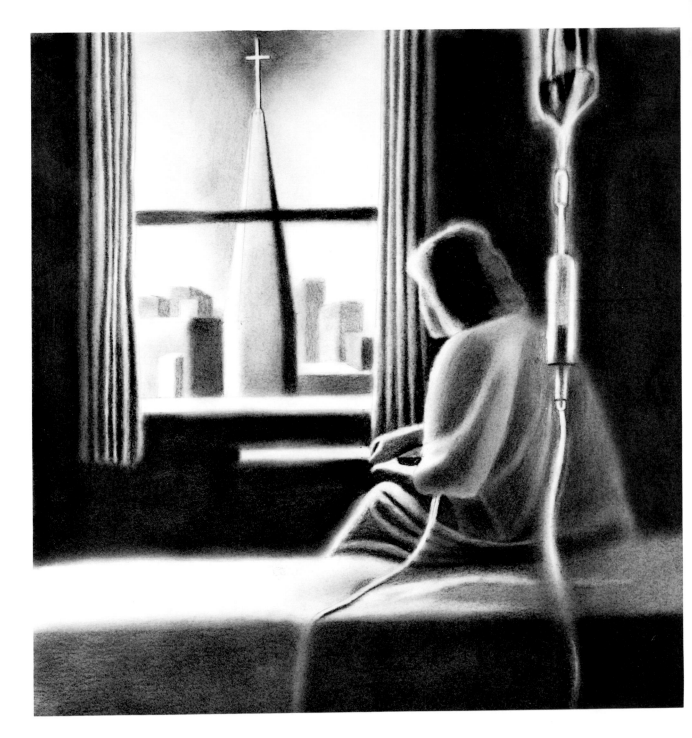

Steeple

I spent a number of weeks at the Princess Margaret Hospital in Toronto, where I received radiation treatments to my abdomen, overseen by Dr. Simon Sutcliffe. While there, I noticed there was a church, Our Lady of Lourdes, next to the hospital. Later I returned to conduct research for this art project. When interviewing a patient, I again noticed the church through the window and got the idea for this image.

In terms of form, the vertical thrust of the steeple and the IV bag echo each other. As well, they both shine with light. The drawing is deliberately ambiguous. The steeple could be a symbol of salvation, a beacon of meaning in a meaningless situation. Or, conversely, the steeple could be read as an impotent icon, useless and unreachable, sealed off outside the window of the modern scientific world. The woman sits in a darkened room, suspended between these poles.

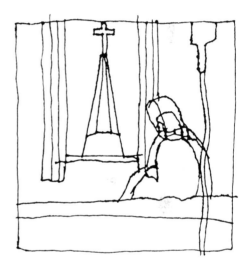

Above:
Steeple, 1990
Ink on paper, 4.8 x 4.8 cm

Opposite:
Steeple, 1990
Charcoal on paper, 32.4 x 32.4 cm

93

Listening

One afternoon, in talking about the ideas behind this image with my parents, my mother reminded me of the saying that there are no atheists in foxholes. In cancer, many of the cases end in death despite the intervention of modern medicine. This not only tends to shake people's faith in science, but opens the possibility of an experience beyond the physical. Often cancer forces the patient to raise his consciousness, a positive thing. An increased spirituality can be very useful on a practical level when faced with a difficult circumstance.

In this scheme of things, the role of the chaplain becomes as important, or more important, than that of the physician. I was inspired to attempt a picture involving a chaplain after seeing a photograph of a mass for terminal patients taking place at St. Rose's Home, run by Hawthorne Dominicans for the care of incurable cancer patients, in New York City. When I approached Ed Fiander, an Anglican chaplain in Halifax, about doing something similar, he was somewhat negative. He explained how his work consisted mainly in intimate, one-on-one visits with patients rather than more public rituals with fancy vestments.

After this conversation, I decided to proceed with two images: *Service for Terminal Patients* and *Listening*, and I believe Rev. Fiander's criticisms were valid. *Service for Terminal Patients* comes off as a bizarre mix of 1930s social realism and Dickensian melodrama. *Listening* seems more successful, with its themes of awareness, and communication on more than one level.

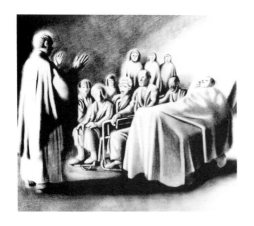

Above:
Service for Terminal Patients, 1990
Charcoal on paper, 35.5 x 41.3 cm

Opposite:
Listening, 1990
Ink on paper, 8.0 x 8.7 cm

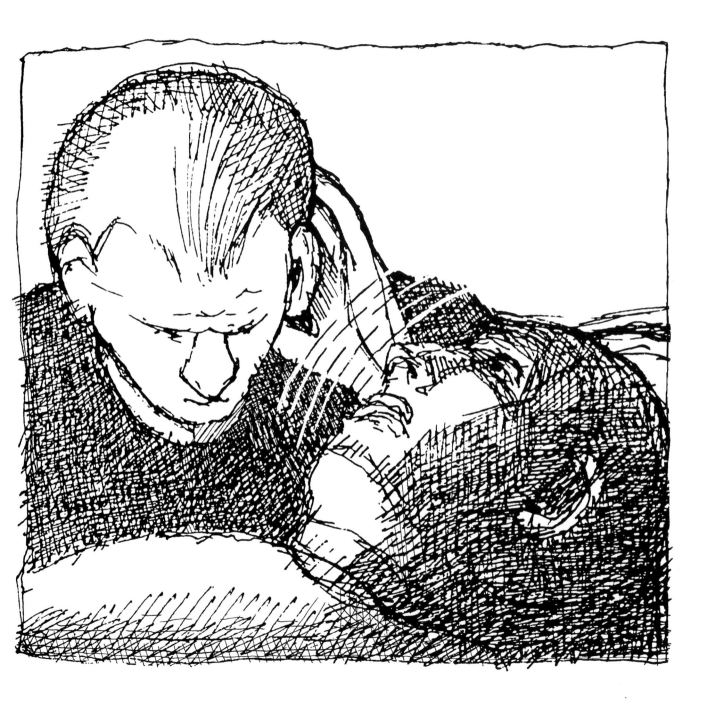

Daughter and Father

As our population ages and more people develop cancer, more sons and daughters will be put in the position of having to care for their parents with the disease. This drawing deals with some of the issues raised by this relationship.

An illness can bring a family closer together, yet difficulties such as difference of age and trouble in adjusting to changing roles can set up stumbling blocks to any new-found closeness. Sometimes the case arises where the sick parent is better able to cope than the healthy offspring.

To suggest these ideas, I placed the daughter and father in different areas of the ink sketch, connected by the umbilical cord of the bed. The father is rendered in an illustrational, crosshatched style, while the daughter is depicted more abstractly in solid blacks and whites. The father looks off to the side, the daughter stares blankly at the viewer, her face like a pagan mask.

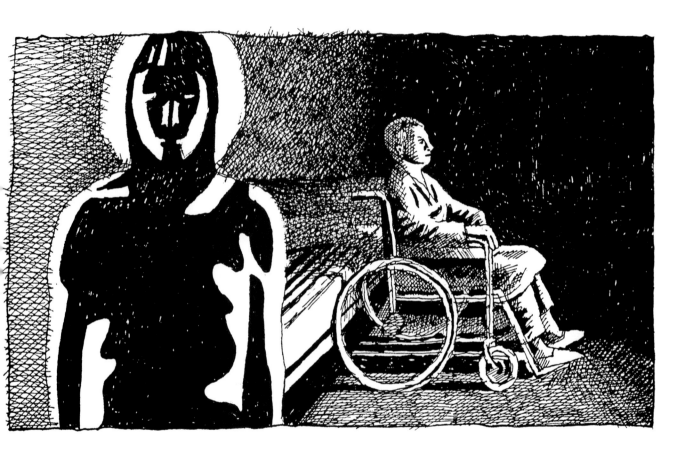

Daughter and Father, 1990
Ink on paper, 10.4 x 18.0 cm

97

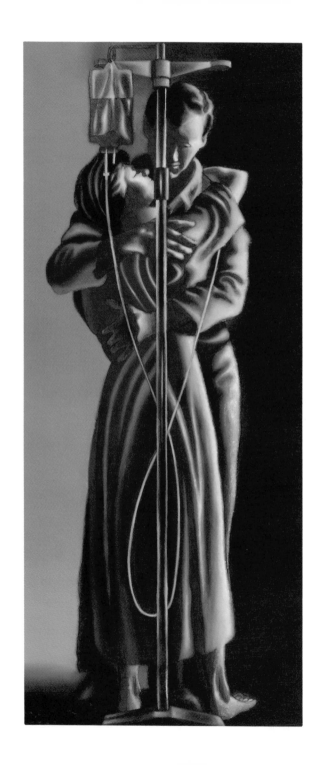

98

Hug

This image was a search for a monumental set of forms that would deal with families coping with cancer. The painting is six feet high and the figures are life-size. It is deceptively simple, but it took me three couples and countless drawings to arrive at the final composition. The two main opposing forces are life and death. The gesture of the hug is life-affirming. The colour grows redder where the figures touch. The IV pole, suggesting a cross, slashes through the couple like a dagger, splitting them in two, a reminder of mortality.

With the content dictating the forms, the people are made up of intertwining curves, while the IV pole is made of straight lines. The formal tension mirrors the psychological tension. I worked wet in wet with a feathery blending brush to evoke a sense of fluidity. The folds of the clothing, the anatomy of the figures, even the cord of the IV bag are manipulated to create a spiralling rhythm. Man, woman, life, and death melt together. In this spiral of forms and ideas I have tried to find a compassionate equivalent for the struggle cancer patients and their loved ones go through.

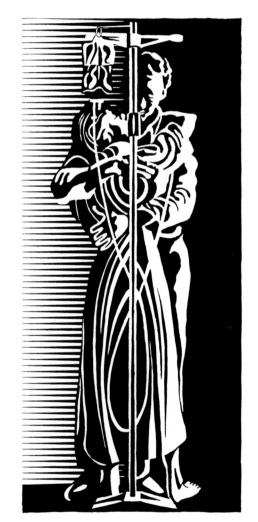

Left:
Hug, 1990
Acrylic on canvas, 182.9 x 78.7 cm

This page:
Hug, 1990
Ink on paper, 41.2 x 18.9 cm

Mastectomy

One of the most disturbing aspects of cancer treatment is that it sometimes involves amputation. As humans, we desire a sense of completeness, and with the loss of a body part, this feeling is disrupted. Canada's most well known cancer amputee is Terry Fox. He demonstrated very convincingly that the loss of a leg need not slow him down, nor anyone else.

This image deals with the theme of a mastectomy — the surgical removal of a breast to prevent the spread of cancer. As a man I am not sure I can fully understand all the feelings associated with this procedure, but I am sure it must be very difficult to cope with. In our fragmented society, where body parts are isolated and arranged in a hierarchy of importance defined by the culture, the loss of a breast becomes a worst case scenario.

In talking this over with several female friends, a number of points were raised. There is a sense of violation and a feeling of being less of a woman. There is the worry that a mastectomy will change the relationship between the woman and her male partner, sexually and otherwise. In the end, however, one friend put this in its proper perspective. She reminded me that a man should be very grateful that his partner is still alive, by far the most important fact.

Opposite:
Mastectomy, 1991
Ink on paper, 10.5 x 11.5 cm

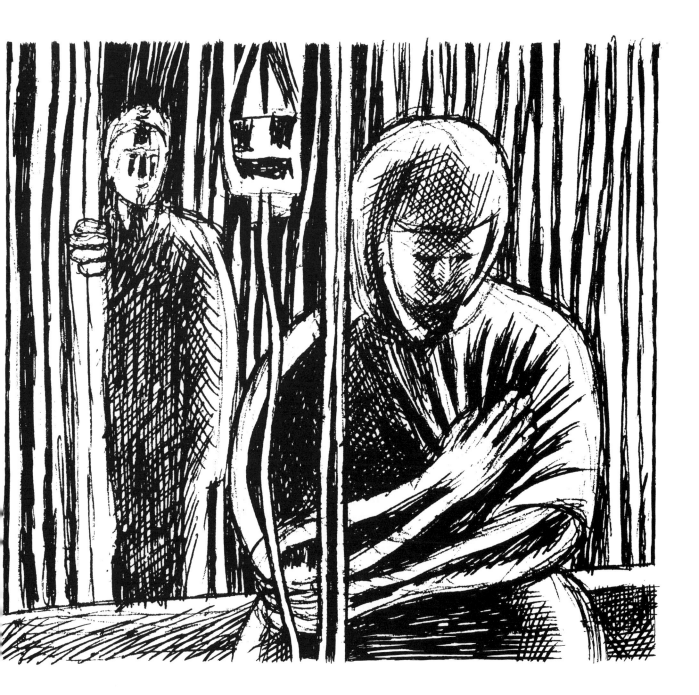

Progress

The models for the standing people in this drawing are Terry Blakeney, a friend since boyhood, and his family. My studio is small, and things got rather chaotic as three adults and three lively children tried to work out a complicated pose at extremely close quarters. At times during the session, I felt as though I were in a Marx Brothers movie, and I am sure Terry and the others must have considered the situation equally preposterous.

Progress, which occupied me for an entire autumn, is a multi-generational group of figures exploring family relationships, illness, and health. It looks back at the past and forward to the future. It is stacked with symbols that spiral and fold into one another.

The figures are arranged on a vertical axis, creating the effect of a totem pole. At the top is the ubiquitous television, its blank, blind white screen presiding like a mindless electronic god. Moving down, we notice the cancer-stricken grandfather, lying prone in bed. Next is the father who looks toward the patient. The mother, lost in thought, gazes sideways as she holds her daughter. This girl looks through a telescope, representing an attempt to see the future. Continuing down, we come to the first boy, holding a hand of cards, a symbol of chance, or fate. Finally we arrive at the youngest boy, playing with an oxygen mask, alluding to pollution and the world's environmental crisis.

This image can be likened to a cautionary parable. It reminds us of negative aspects of life: blindness, sickness, pollution. Yet this spiral of figures also suggests that hope and health can be achieved through human solidarity and the establishment of a vision for the future.

Opposite:
Progress, 1991
Acrylic on canvas, 182.9 x 121.8 cm

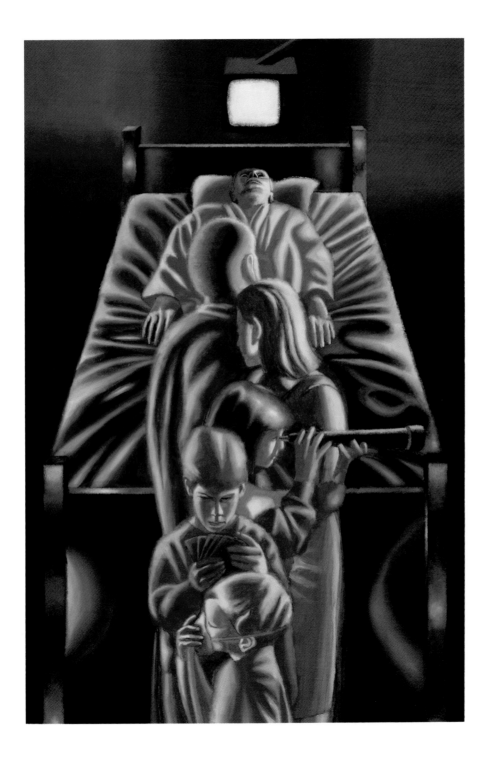

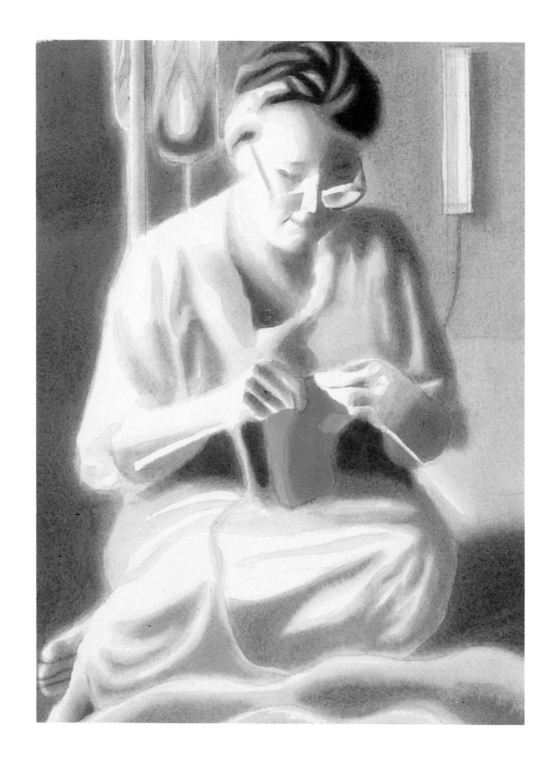

Red Mitten

The notion that prompted me to do this watercolour came about during a visit with a cancer patient in Toronto. The woman, who owned and operated a successful doll-making business, was knitting a red mitten. This struck me as a wonderfully positive, and Canadian, symbol.

Everything but this element is painted in whites and greys. As is often the case, the symbolic key to my picture is placed in the physical center. At this focal point of the composition, near the woman's heart, the mitten is a bright red. It evokes feelings of life, warmth, and survival.

Opposite:
Red Mitten, 1989
Acrylic on paper, 34.5 x 25.8 cm

Mrs. Oochigeaskw

Often my pictures are a fusion of radically different sources. In this case, aspects of two real women are combined with a memory of my own experience.

For a long time I had wanted to do an image of a patient in a hospital hallway. I remember late night hours when, agitated by drugs, I would endlessly pace the deserted, gleaming corridors.

This pencil drawing is partly based on a Micmac woman I met. I have given her the name Mrs. Oochigeaskw which is Micmac for "She Who Is Covered With Scars." There is a contrast between the geometric emptiness of the background and her organic, human presence.

The deeper spirit of this image, however, draws from my memories of my friend Beulah Murphy, who recently died of cancer after a long battle with the disease. I have never met a more strong-willed person, and her life-force was a source of wonder. I will always think of her standing straight up, resolute in the face of hardship.

Opposite:
Mrs. Oochigeaskw, 1990
Pencil on paper, 17.0 x 17.0 cm

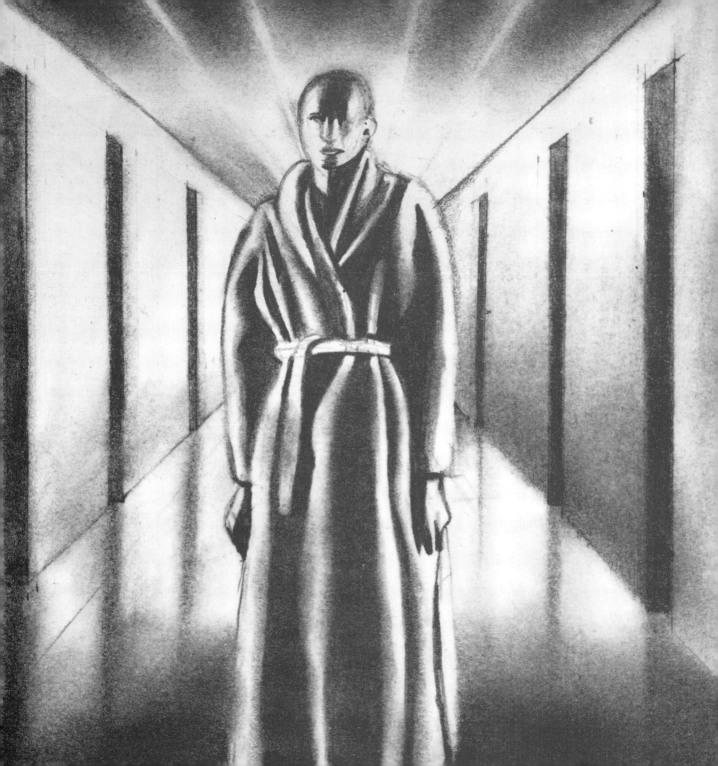

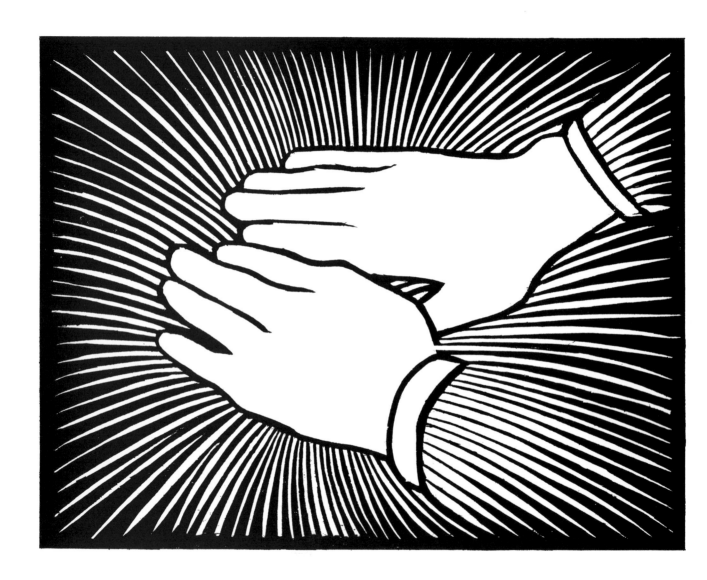

Healing Hands

For several years I shared a studio with Glen Mac-Kinnon, a gifted artist who has created many striking woodcuts. With his encouragement, and technical assistance, I attempted my first woodcut, and *Healing Hands* is the result.

The human body seems to have an innate ability to heal. One aspect of healing is the involvement of touch. When we have a headache, we place our hand on our forehead. When we have a sore shoulder, we rub it. When someone we love is in pain, we hold them.

Previously, I had done a watercolour version of this image in soft flesh tones. In this woodcut, the additional device of the lines radiating from the hands increases the graphic interest and serves to convey a sense of healing power. The lines symbolize curative life energy flowing inside and outside the body.

Below:
Healing Hands, 1989
Ink on paper, 5.5 x 7.0 cm

Opposite:
Healing Hands, 1989
Woodcut, 25.4 x 33.0 cm

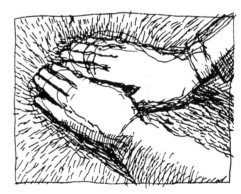

Curtain

As an artist, I find I have two distinct audiences. One group is a public one, comprised of people I do not know. The second audience is a smaller, more intimate circle made up of those I am closer to: they are nearer to the creative process and see the work more regularly.

One member of this second group is my brother, Doug. He frequently will offer painting ideas to me and, indeed, bemoans the fact that I don't follow his suggestions more often. He is quite interested in a theme common in nineteenth century literature, that of "the double," as can be seen in such stories as Edgar Allen Poe's *William Wilson*. One day as I was showing Doug a half worked out sketch of a man lying in bed, he suggested adding a curtain and putting a second man on the other side, thus making the image more psychological and evocative.

This painting recalls memories of lying in bed in the hospital with a curtain drawn between my neighbour and myself. Even though I couldn't see the man in the next bed, I would be very conscious of his presence, a rather dissimilar feeling to being alone in a room.

In this picture, the two men are painted very differently. The light on the man in the foreground produces a sense of volume, whereas the backlighting of the other man turns him into a flat silhouette. This, coupled with the separation of the curtain, implies that each man could be symbolic of a different state: healing and illness, life and death. Or, in keeping with my brother's notion, this picture could represent opposite sides of the same person.

Opposite:
Curtain, 1990
Acrylic on canvas, 61.0 x 61.0 cm

110

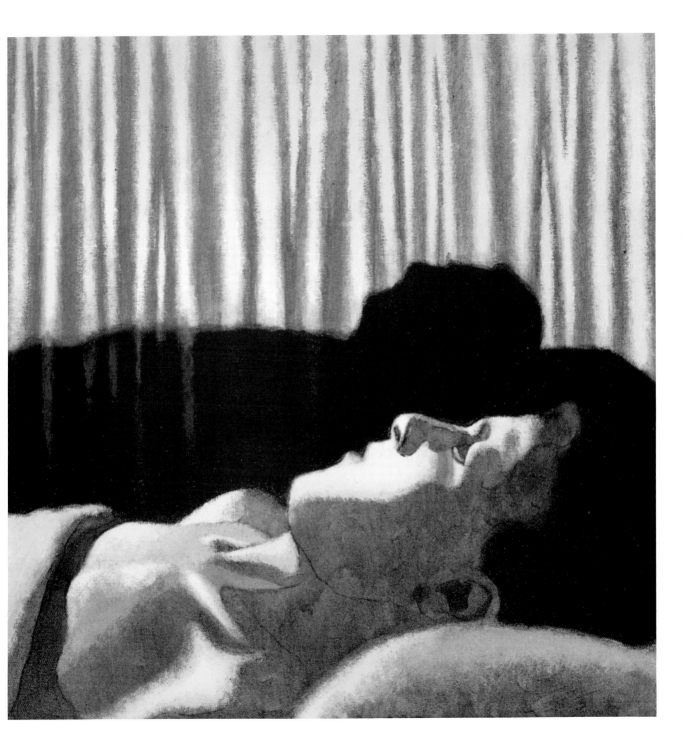

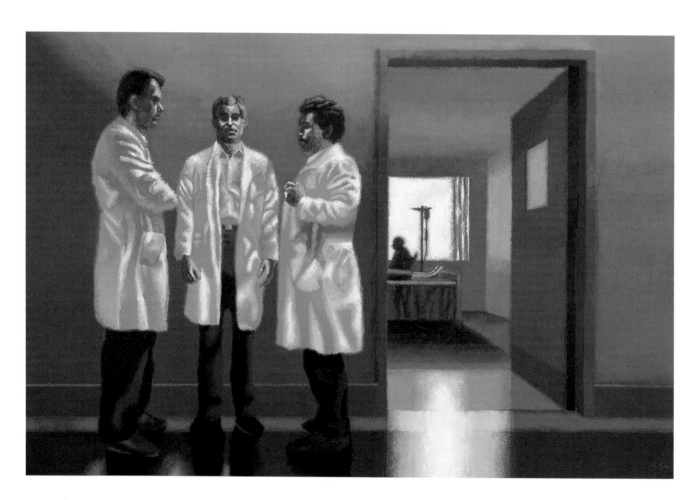

Conference

This painting, like the drawing *A Friend's Story*, contrasts events in a hallway with what is happening in an adjoining room. A group of three doctors are having a discussion outside the room, while inside we see a patient lying in bed, and a visitor.

I wanted this painting to be about the subtleties of communication and exchange of information in a cancer situation: doctors talk differently among themselves than they do to the patient or the family. In the hall the language is scientific, factual and blunt; meanwhile, in the room the communication is of a more nurturing and emotional nature. I based the composition for this painting on another painting about privilege and lack of it: *The Flagellation of Christ* by Piero Della Francesco.

Opposite:
Conference, 1990
Acrylic on canvas, 61.0 x 91.4 cm

Family

Below:
Family, 1990
Ink on paper, 10.9 x 14.2 cm

Opposite:
Family, 1990
Acrylic on canvas, 91.4 x 121.9 cm

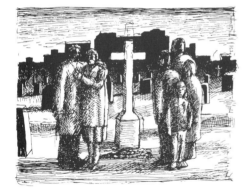

I was trying to do three things in this big, dense painting about death. The first was to create a set of symbols. Second, I wanted to explore the psychological reactions and interrelationships of the family members. Third, I wanted to set the people in a social context, relating them to their human and cultural environment.

The Victoria General Hospital and the cemetery are physical structures and are symbols of rationality and order. The cross, representing another type of order, has obvious symbolism. The dog in the foreground, added to the painting last, is the key to the image. Occupying the center of the picture like a black hole, the dog's raw emotional intensity unsettles the static structure of the other elements. It can be read as a symbol of the natural world, of rage, of sorrow, or as a dark side of spirituality, rising from hidden recesses. One friend who was hoping this would be a nice, Christian picture was very disturbed by the inclusion of the dog.

There are a series of interior dialogues set up by contrasting pairings within the image. The howling of the dog is juxtaposed with the man holding the saxophone. On the left, the man looks toward the grave, while his wife looks away. This couple is in turn contrasted to the group at the right of the grave. Finally, and perhaps summarizing the painting, the only pairs of eyes that engage the viewer are those of the girl in the foreground and the dog.

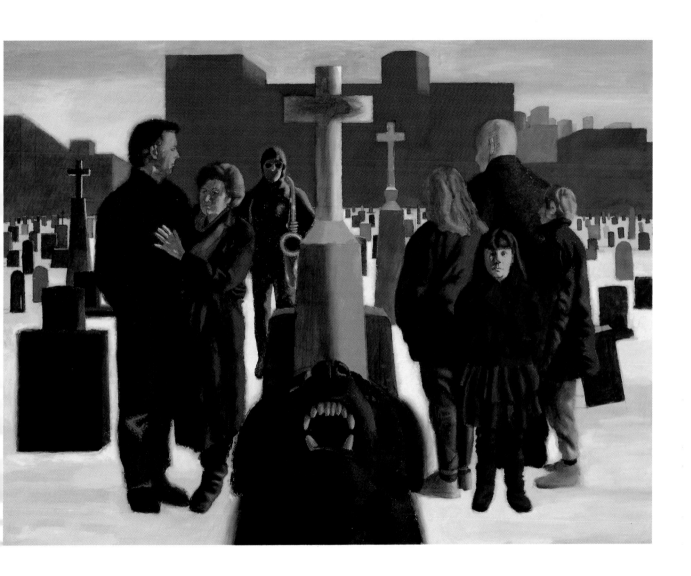

The Gift

When in Toronto gathering background material for this project, I had the opportunity to go through the photo file of the public relations department of the Princess Margaret Hospital. One of the most memorable photographs was of a young father holding a baby. The father's hair had fallen out as a result of chemotherapy; I wanted to use this image of baldness to contrast how the baby is experiencing new life while the man is confronting the potential end of life.

My picture didn't seem complete until I added the figure of the mother, making the theme of fertility more explicit. My sister calls it a "malignant holy family." When I was given chemotherapy, the doctor told me the treatment would cause sterility, a side effect that has been very difficult to accept and deal with. This image is of a minor miracle then, birth occurring in the life of a chemotherapy patient, hinting that he too may live.

I chose the title *The Gift* for two reasons. One reason is that the birth of a child is like a gift to the parents. The other reason is that after a serious illness, life itself is experienced as the greatest gift any person can receive.

Opposite:
The Gift, 1991
Acrylic on canvas, 22.9 x 30.5 cm

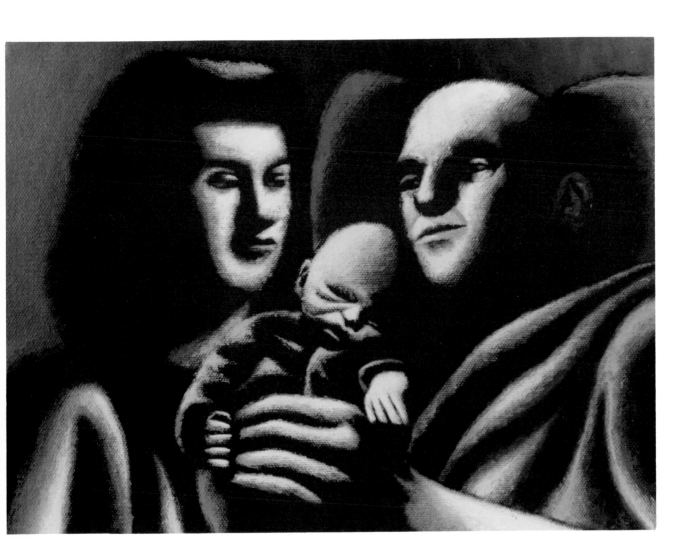

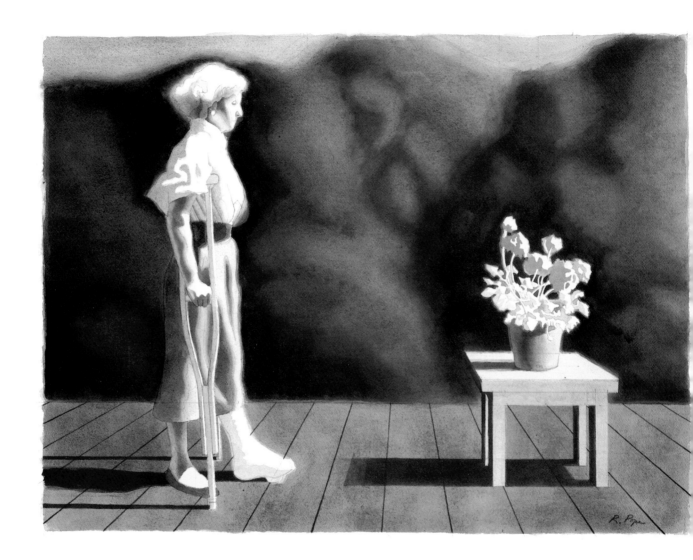

The First Day

This image was created about one third of the way into my series. A friend, Mary Cutler, who is a nurse, commented at the time that this painting was a breakthrough in that it was the first picture in the project that directly dealt with healing.

At one stage in the process of getting better, I recall sitting on the deck of my parents' house and noticing a pot of geraniums. It was mid-morning in early summer. The flowers seemed to be gloriously alive in the bright, warm sunlight. Ordinary as this may seem, this has somehow remained a watershed moment for me. The picture records those strong impressions: the deck, the geraniums, the sunlight, and the act of contemplation.

Sickness, I believe, carries with it thoughts of possibilities being closed off, of senses being shut down, of feelings of reluctance in engaging with the world. Health, in contrast, involves an expansion of possibilities, and an opening-up cycle that might be likened to a blossom unfolding in the warmth of the sun.

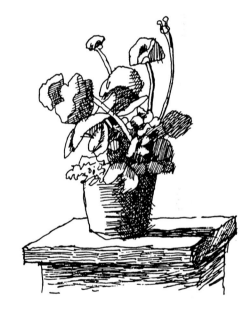

Above:
Geraniums, 1989
Ink on paper, 10.0 x 8.5 cm

Opposite:
The First Day, 1989
Acrylic on paper, 53.5 x 71.8 cm

119

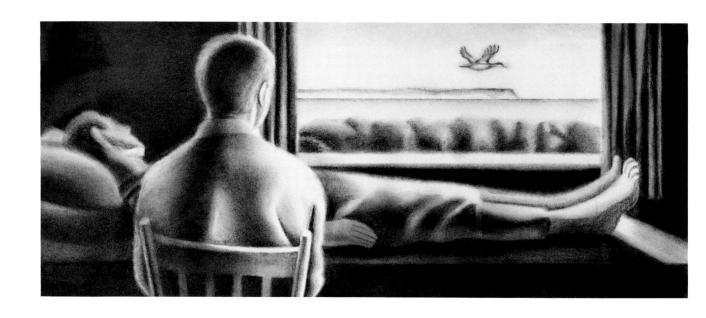

Brothers

While recovering from cancer, much of my time was
spent in a bedroom in my parent's house in the
Annapolis Valley. Apples are the main crop of this rich,
lush farming area and I have always looked on the
valley as a sort of earthly paradise. From this period my
clearest recollections are the presence of my family and
the view from my bedroom window.

Through the window can be seen tree tops, the Bay
of Fundy, and rising above everything else, the long
mountain ridge that ends in Cape Blomidon. In Micmac
culture, Blomidon is the home of their god, Glooscap, a
mythic idea that reinforced my feeling of a spiritualized
landscape.

A bird passes by the window in the picture. It
suggests flight, passage, progress; perhaps the person in
bed may likewise move on soon and begin to get well.
The title is meant to imply that in a healthy world there
is a relatedness on earth, a kinship that connects the
trees, the bird, the water, the mountain, the sky and the
men.

Opposite:
Brothers, 1991
Charcoal on paper, 16.1 x 39.7 cm

New Steps

This art project would not have been possible without the help of nurses. I have been working mainly with the same group of women who nursed me when I was sick. The picture *New Steps* came out of a conversation I had with Gloria Repetto and Janet Copeland, whose assistance has been invaluable. They suggested an image of two nurses walking a patient. I immediately liked the idea because it was active, rather than passive, and it involved cooperation of both parties, as equals. The act of taking new steps could be a metaphor for healing itself.

Earlier versions of *New Steps* included a number of people in the corridor, looking on in amazement as the patient returns like Lazarus to his feet. Realizing that the scene could still be amazing without the spectators, and that a simplified composition would have more impact, I reduced it to the three main figures.

The image evolved even more as I began experimenting with elongating the figures. I noticed that my pictures of illness, with people lying in bed, tend to be horizontal while my images of healing, usually with upright figures, are generally vertical, and began to wonder if there was something about vertical forms that was inherently healing. Here, the nurses and patient rise upward like church architecture or the figures of El Greco. They spring forth like flames in an image of partnership on the walk back to health.

Below:
New Steps, 1990
Charcoal on paper, 34.7 x 39.0 cm

Opposite:
New Steps, 1991
Charcoal on paper, 106.5 x 64.0 cm

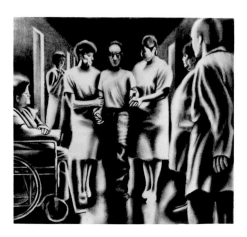

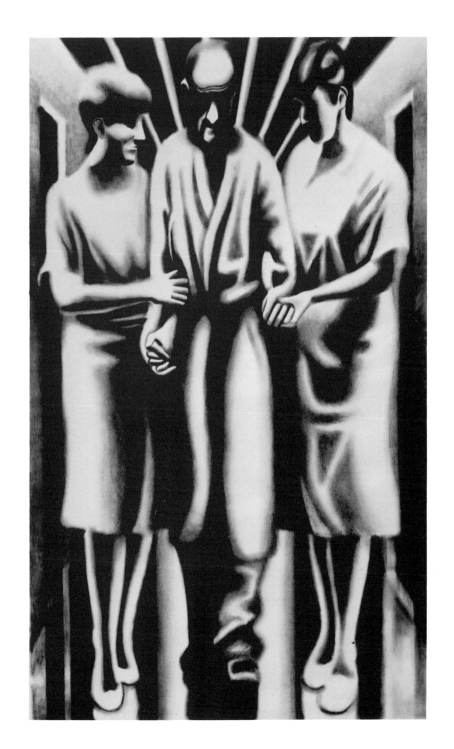

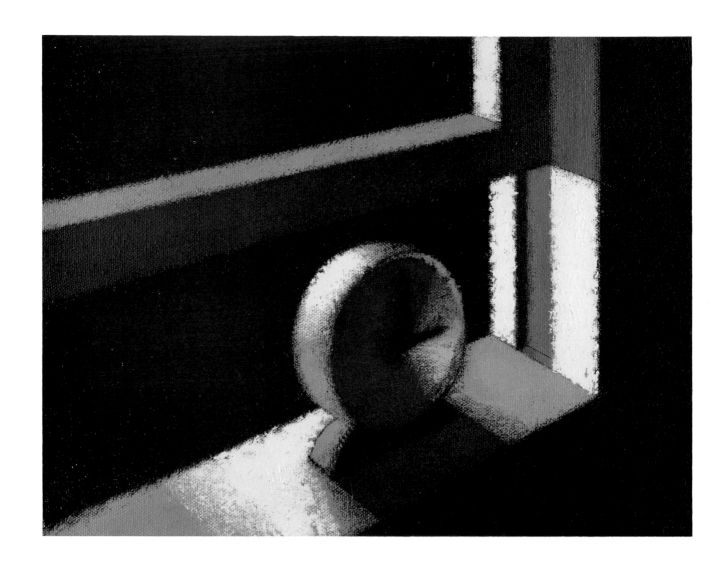

124

Window

Many images in this body of work use the motif of the window. It is a device that allows both inside and outside to be seen together. In several of the pictures the window carries with it psychological and metaphorical connotations. The view through the window becomes a vista into the mind, or a spiritual dimension. That is especially the case with this cosmic little drawing.

I had been haunted by the concept of an open window for some time before doing this image. It symbolizes to me a passageway to a new, perhaps spiritual, world and a sense of release, or freedom. I also saw an open window as representing an open mind. I deliberately left the view outside the window empty: what I wanted was a feeling of infinity.

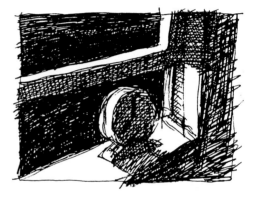

Above:
Clock in Window, Night, 1989
Ink on paper, 5.0 x 6.5 cm

Opposite:
Window, 1991
Acrylic on canvas, 22.9 x 30.5 cm

Illness and Healing

Themes of illness and healing, from which this book draws its title, are restated and fused here. This image depicts a family visiting in the hospital. Silhouetted against the window is a solitary figure, signifying isolation, darkness, illness and death. In the front, an adult and child embrace, representing togetherness, love, health, and life.

The patient is placed between these two symbols. It remains to be seen in which direction he will move. Meanwhile, he lies in bed, the candle keeping vigil beside him.

Opposite:
Illness and Healing, 1991
Ink on board, 14.3 x 18.1 cm

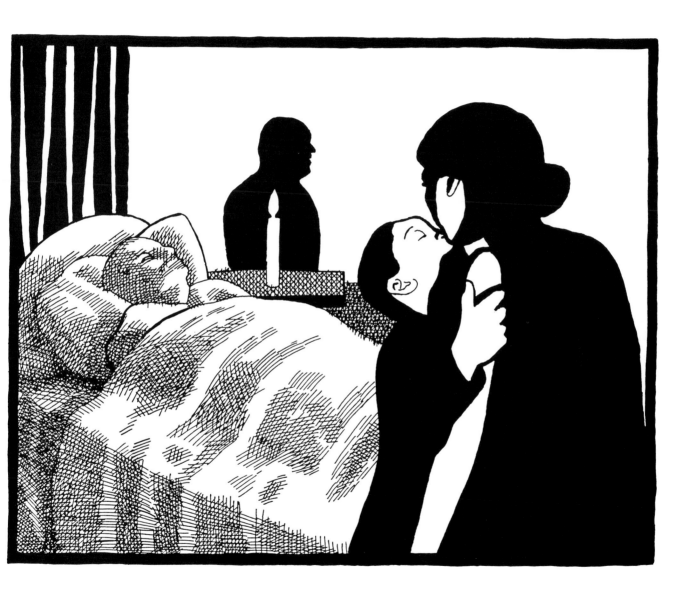

Sink

Sink examines the relationship within a marriage in which one of the partners has cancer. I purposely left it unclear as to whether the husband or wife is ill. To me, it could be the husband, but most people see the wife as being the one with cancer here.

The couple share the same bed, but they do not share the same thoughts. The husband sleeps while his wife lies awake, staring upward, her mind racing. Echoing her rushing thoughts is the stream of water flowing from the tap in the background. I understand the sink in two ways: first, the moving water as a symbol of life, and second, the drain as a metaphor for life slipping away. The man's hand is cupped in an upcast direction, in a gesture of catching the water, or holding onto life.

Again, I have reduced the elements of the image to the bare essentials. On one level I wanted this picture to be quite realistic, dealing with some disturbing actualities. On another level, however, it seems to resonate poetically.

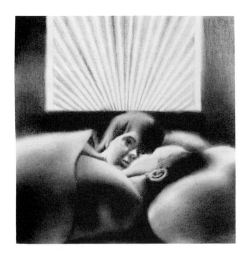

Above:
Sunrise, 1991
Charcoal on paper, 35.0 x 35.0 cm

Opposite:
Sink, 1990
Charcoal on paper, 35.5 x 36.0 cm

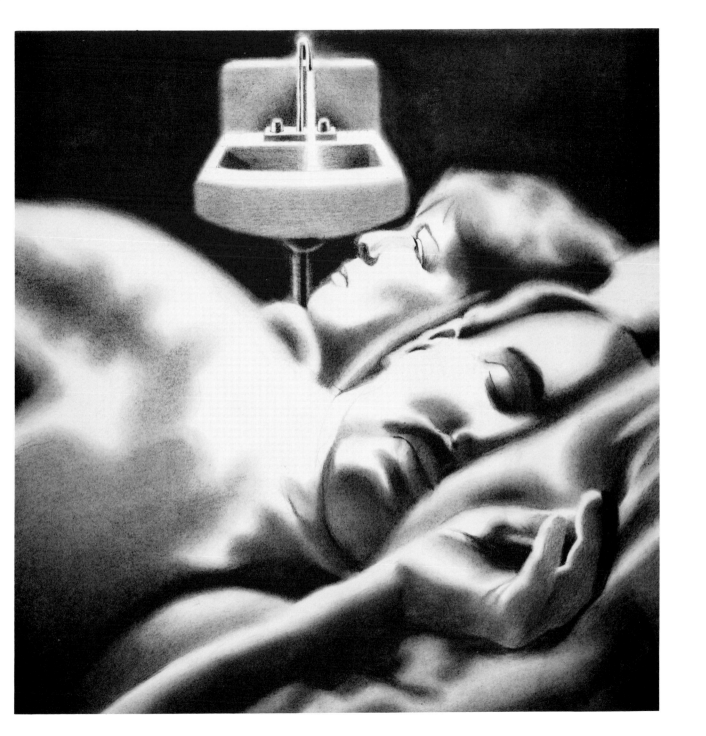

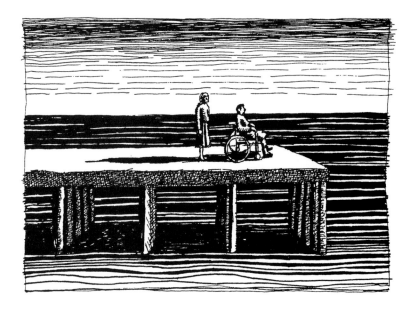

This page:
Healing, 1990
Ink on paper, 12.0 x 16.8 cm

Opposite:
Healing, 1990
Acrylic on canvas, 61.0 x 91.4 cm

Healing

The studio in which I work is on the waterfront, very close to a wharf, and I have used this motif many times. For me, contemporary life is being lived increasingly on the edge. This is especially true for cancer patients, most of whom face a real uncertainty whether they will live or die. The wharf, which is on the physical edge of land and water, seemed an apt metaphor for this psychological reality.

This journey to the edge of death is a difficult thing to face, and I am amazed by the courage most cancer patients show. In this image, with someone to stand by him, a man sits in a wheelchair at the end of a wharf. The wharf becomes a stage. The man and his companion are bathed in golden sunlight, participants in a drama of healing.

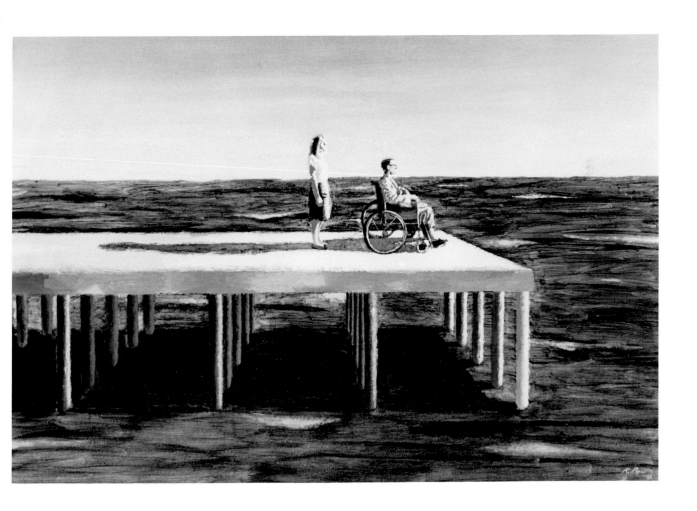

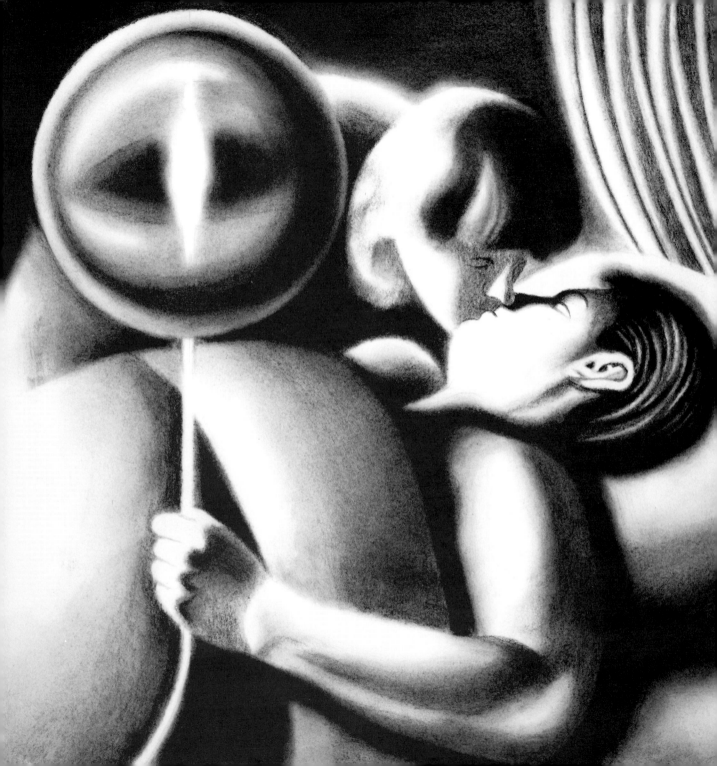

Balloon

The germination of this image came about one day in the office of my doctor, Ross Langley. I was showing him what I had done so far and he commented that I had far more pictures of illness than of healing. I asked him if he could suggest anything, and after a mini-brainstorming session, the notion of a party given to celebrate the end of chemotherapy was put forward. This work finally came together when I saw a photograph of two well-known Mexican artists: Diego Rivera bending over the bed to kiss his sick wife, Frida Kahlo.

Formally, I wanted this drawing to be composed entirely of curves and rounded shapes. The balloon of the title is a metallic, helium filled type, a common gift to patients. Here, it is a symbol of celebration. As the man and the woman kiss, we notice the vague reflection of a nurse in the balloon. She overlooks the scene like a guardian angel.

Opposite:
Balloon, 1990
Charcoal on paper, 35.6 x 35.6 cm

New Field

This small watercolour is one of the few works in this book that does not contain a human figure, although a nearby human presence is implied. The field of wheat is a symbol of life. In fact, wheat is known as the staff of life. It, and other grains such as rice and corn, have been absolutely central to human development.

In the foreground lies a pair of crutches, a symbol of illness. Health has returned, and the crutches, once so important, are no longer needed. The patient has walked out of the picture, and gets on with life.

In discussions with Susan Gibson Garvey, curator at the Dalhousie Art Gallery, she commented on the sense of enclosure and claustrophobia in much of this body of work. This touches on one of the central differences between illness and health. Illness is largely self-absorption. The patient is not aware of much beyond his or her bed. Most healthy persons are concerned with a larger world: interests, friends, their work, and the physical environment that surrounds them.

The images in this book are sequenced so they loosely move from illness to healing, and from claustrophobia to openness. As the book progresses, we get more and more glimpses out of windows, then we see people outdoors, and finally with this image we are presented with a pure landscape.

Opposite:
New Field, 1989
Acrylic on paper, 25.0 x 34.0 cm

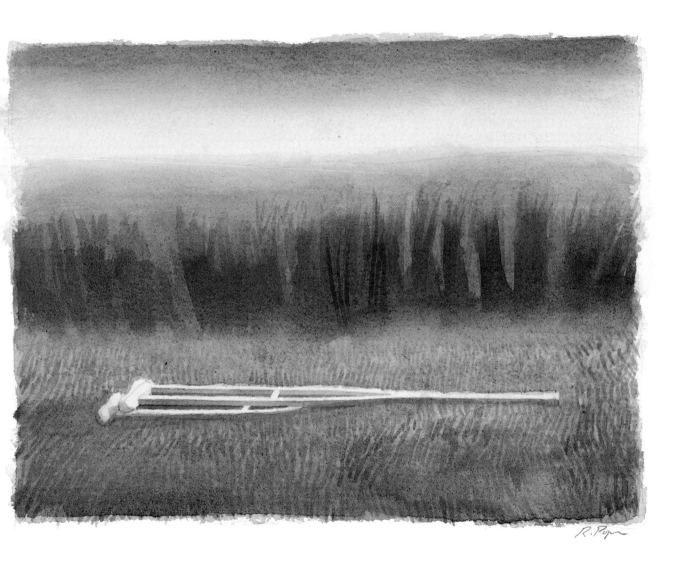

Photograph Credits

All colour photographs are by Steve Zwerling
Photography Limited. David Miller took the
photographs on pages 22, 29, 43, 49, 53, 79, 86, 90, 94,
111, 112, 117, 124, and 131. All other photographs are
by Doug Pope.

Note on Prevention

The present consensus is that the vast majority of all cancer is preventable. The following list, approved by the Canadian Cancer Society, provides a basis for personal actions which may reduce your risk of cancer.

1. Eat a high fibre diet. High fibre foods include: porridge, cereal, bread, pasta, rice, and beans (lentils, chick peas, navy beans, etc.).
2. Have several servings of vegetables and fruit daily.
3. Maintain a low total fat intake. Fat comes in many forms — as visible fat on meat and poultry, as hidden fat in dairy products, in baked goods, or as added fat in rich sauces, gravy, butter, or oil.
4. Avoid consumption of smoked, nitrate-cured, highly salted or charred foods.
5. Keep your weight close to ideal.
6. Minimize or eliminate alcohol.
7. Do not smoke.
8. Avoid radiation, including excessive sunlight and non-essential x-rays.
9. Avoid occupations that involve exposure to known carcinogens.
10. Exercise regularly.
11. Maintain good relationships with your family and friends. Open up. Share your feelings with others. Hug someone you care about, every day.
12. Be relaxed. Deep breathing, exercising, and relaxation techniques all help.

There are many ways to incorporate the suggestions on the previous page into your lifestyle. Personally, I follow a macrobiotic program which includes all aspects of this list. Macrobiotics, which means "great life," has been of benefit to many cancer patients as well as offering health improvement to anyone. For further information contact:

Macrobiotics Canada
RR3 Almonte, Ont.
K0A 1A0
(613) 256-2665

List of Full-Page Images

About the Author

Robert Pope was born in Halifax, Nova Scotia in 1956. The son of a United Church minister and a bookkeeper, he grew up in several small towns throughout the province, spending his teenage years in Windsor, Nova Scotia. He was educated at Acadia University in Wolfville, where he received a Bachelor of Science degree in 1977, and the Nova Scotia College of Art and Design in Halifax, where he graduated with a Bachelor of Fine Arts degree in 1981.

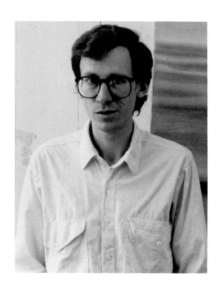

In 1982 he was diagnosed with cancer, and received treatment in Halifax and Toronto off and on for the next five years. Also during this decade, his art began to be exhibited in numerous group shows across Canada.

His solo exhibitions have included *A Seal Upon Thine Heart* at Saint Mary's University Art Gallery in 1988 and *Accident* at Studio 21 in 1989. He was awarded Canada Council grants in 1989 and 1990 that enabled him to work full-time on the *Illness and Healing* project, exhibited at the Dalhousie Art Gallery in 1991.